HOW MY BREASTS SAVED THE WORLD

Lisa Wood Shapiro

Misadventures

of a Nursing Mother

HOW MY BREASTS SAVED THE WORLD

THE LYONS PRESS / Guilford, Connecticut

An imprint of The Globe Pequot Press

To buy books in quantity for corporate use
or incentives, call **(800) 962–0973, ext. 4551,**
or e-mail **premiums@GlobePequot.com.**

FOR SOPHIE, EBEN, AND PETER

Contents

Preface

The Most Natural Thing in the World and Brooke Shields

THE WOMEN in my family held certain convictions that they believed to be true. They thought women and girls looked best in short pixie haircuts, and this misconception was imposed on their daughters at random. They believed one could never own enough cookbooks, a game of bridge was good for the soul, and that women should breast-feed their babies.

"Breast-feeding is the most natural thing in the world," my grandmother used to say. "Why would anyone do anything else?" My grandmother wasn't one for keeping her opinions to herself and she was more confounded than judgmental when it came to nursing. She didn't own a dishwasher until in her forties and couldn't understand why anyone would clean all those bottles and boil all those nipples.

I cannot say when I was conscious of the fact that my family came from a long line of breast-feeders—I mean didn't we all—but my family kept on nursing even after the advent of formula and the trend toward prop feeding. They were proud of this and though they weren't the kind of people who bragged, they flaunted this fact whenever the subject of babies came up, which was often.

When I was a child I loved visiting my grandmother who lived in St. Thomas, Virgin Islands. I remember lingering over breakfasts at the kitchen table where we ate fresh papaya and mango. I listened to stories about my mother's childhood. She was eleven when her parents, brother, and sister all relocated to the island. For the first year they lived in a hut on the beach. A colossal resort sits there today, but back in the fifties it was just a one-room beach cabin. My mom ate fresh coconut from the tree and she had several frightening encounters with barracudas. It all was far more exotic than New Jersey, where I grew up. I used to think the only exciting thing that happened to me was being born on that island.

How I came to be born in St. Thomas is a complicated story that involved my parents' meeting at George Washington University, a chicken farm in South Africa, a denial for a renewed visa, and my mother being six months pregnant. But how I was born became part of my family's oral history, usually told every time we visited my grandmother. It was 1969 and my mother was twenty-three years old. My parents left South Africa, where they'd been living, under adverse circumstances. They decided it was best for my mother and sister to live temporarily with my grandparents while my father secured a job up in the States.

I was my mother's second child, due a brief sixteen months after her first. As the story went, after my mother's water broke, my grandmother dropped her off at the front entrance of the hospital. She entered unaccompanied, and she stresses that it was a different time back then, especially in an out-of-the-way Caribbean hospital. Women rarely brought their spouses into the delivery room, much less their mothers. My mother was given an intravenous drip of Pitocin without any pain medication and left alone in the delivery room. There was no one to hold her hand, no nurse to wipe her brow. It was just my mother and Pitocin.

The doctor returned when it came time to push. My mother had given birth to my sister in South Africa with only Demerol to dull the pain, so in her mind she knew she could do it, and she did. Perhaps it's because that story was retold so many times, or it was the only testimonial I ever intimately knew, but either way that story shaped my own perceptions of labor and delivery. It was scary and painful, and one needed to have an advocate and most of all be prepared. That was the hard part.

After the delivery my mom was rolled into the recovery room and I was placed in the hospital's nursery. No longer in pain, she was thrilled to be served hot porridge with raisins, my mother's favorite. Several bites later, my mom noticed that the raisins began to move. They weren't raisins.

"Get me out of here," my mother told my grandma over the phone. She got dressed, got her baby, and walked out of the hospital fourteen hours after giving birth. Since she hadn't been properly discharged she would have to return later for my birth certificate, which in keeping with the hospital's standard of care had listed me as a "male." My mother reapplied for a new certificate with the proper sex, but somewhere in a shoe box of childhood mementos is a birth certificate with my name on it. In front of the typed word "male" my father wrote an "FE" with a blue ballpoint pen.

The story continued with a disputed ending, which has my mother returning to the house just in time to cook for my grandmother's bridge party. With each telling the number of guests grew and my mother described something like a sit-down dinner, which was plausible.

My mother nursed me at my grandmother's house. She was feeding me in the back bedroom when my sister Anne walked in. She looked at me, who was nursing, looked back at my mother, and walked over mouth agape. There was Anne with all her pointy baby teeth moving in to nurse as well. Anne had been weaned long before and my mother didn't want to encourage her to start again.

"'No, no, no,' I told her." My mom would then pretend to protect herself from the canines of an invisible toddler.

"What I loved most about nursing was being in sync," my mother told me. "I would feel my milk come down and at that moment I would hear you cry." She described the time when I was a baby with such pleasure.

For as often as I heard my family's stories about breast-feeding, I had never actually seen anyone nurse. And then I saw *The Blue Lagoon.*

I'm not exactly sure when I first saw the movie, but somewhere between my Bat Mitzvah and high school graduation I had seen *The Blue Lagoon* at least a dozen times.

The movie told the story of two shipwrecked children who blossom into early adulthood and fall in love. I was curious about sex, so *The Blue Lagoon* with its soft-porn elements gave me glimpses into the unknown. Fourteen-year-old Brooke Shields menstruated, lost her virginity, gave birth, and breast-fed.

After Brooke gives birth in the island's underbrush, the young couple bring their newborn back to their bamboo duplex on the beach. Unsure how to feed their new son they offer him a big piece of papaya, which he rejects. Next they pour some coconut milk into his mouth. The baby wails. Finally, Brooke picks up the infant. As she comforts him in her arms a happy accident occurs. The baby, in the right place at the right time, takes hold of her nipple and nurses. We don't see much of the mechanics of breast-feeding, but it looked fairly easy. Brooke wore special pasties and her body double, who was also the film's caterer, was used for the close-up, but you mostly see the back of the baby's head. Later in one of the film's freakier scenes, Christopher Atkins nurses as well, but that's for another book.

I could relate to *The Blue Lagoon.* I was born in the tropics and liked to think of myself as the castaway type.

The thing was, and I should have known this, *The Blue Lagoon* wasn't that realistic. I mean how did they keep all their whites white? And where did she get her nails done, they were beautifully manicured and she opened all those coconuts? And why did I think that nursing scene with Brooke Shields could ever have been close to accurate?

HOW MY BREASTS SAVED THE WORLD

Part One

THERE WERE some green cocoa-nuts he had gathered the day before close by. He took one, removed the green husk, and opened one of the eyes, making an opening also in the opposite side of the shell. The unfortunate infant sucked ravenously at the nut, filled its stomach with the young cocoa-nut juice, vomited violently, and wailed. Emmeline in despair clasped it to her naked breast, wherefrom, in a moment, it was hanging like a leech. It knew more about babies than they did.

H. DE VERE STACPOOLE
The Blue Lagoon: A Romance

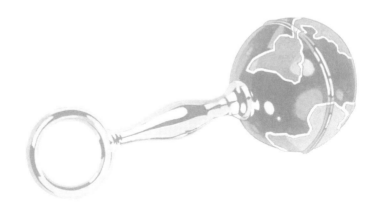

Chapter 1

Silly Pregnant Lady

FOR AS LONG as I can remember, I always wanted children. I participated in the childhood game of asking and telling my girlfriends how many kids we would have and what their names would be. I usually had four imaginary children. Their sex, age, and names changed depending on my mood. There was always one boy named Ivan after an inexplicable crush I had on tennis ace Ivan Lendel. Then there would be twin girls or twin boys followed years later by the youngest, usually named Amanda, nicknamed Mandy after my favorite doll. Money wasn't a consideration. I drew up elaborate floor plans of the homes I would live in. Each child would have his or her own bedroom with a working fireplace and bathroom.

In my teens I remember coming across my old sketch pad. There were pages and pages of those floor plans along with little drawings of each family member. I had taken an art class around that time and knew how to draw a realistic nose. I colored in their hair, giving the girls long locks and boys short curls. I loved sketching twins the most because it was a challenge to do the same figure twice.

After flipping through the pad, I threw the whole thing in the trash without a second's thought. I had outgrown playing pretend when I hit puberty. I had moved on to marching band, boys, and track. The fact that I wasn't particularly talented at any of these was beside the point.

Between the day I threw my make-believe families in the garbage and the day I was ready to start my own, I had been busy. I couldn't wait to graduate high school. I was always anticipating the next step and filling the pages of my photo albums with the evidence of my last. In my northern New Jersey high school yearbook, below my senior photo, is the caption I submitted. It says something snotty like, "Looking forward to leaving *this* town." And I did. I spent several years living in Finland and Israel, moved to Manhattan, went to film school, met a guy, waitressed, worked on films, temped, moved to Brooklyn, got married, worked in television, rode horses, and started a company.

Not long after I turned thirty I began to play that game again, this time with my husband Peter. No longer interested in drawing up fantasy blueprints, I thought up ways to expand our two-bedroom Brooklyn rental. We could turn one walk-in closet into an office with the other becoming a tiny third bedroom. Again I imagined a slew of names for our family-to-be, like Emma, Henry, and Sophie. Little did I know those names were as ubiquitous at our neighborhood playgrounds as pigeons, but that is how it goes for the childless.

Peter and I had been married nearly four years and our trial run with parenthood had gone well: our black Labrador Halley was our first child. Peter proved to be a great dog dad. I, of course, had promised to split the walks fifty/fifty, but somehow it ended up being more like ninety/ten, with Peter doing the ninety. We took Halley on vacations; she was the perfect hiking companion. And we did the queerest of dog-owner things. We celebrated her birthday.

The television production company I had co-founded was doing well. Our reality series about a kid's baseball team was picked up by a children's cable channel. Peter, who worked in publishing as a literary agent, had several large book sales. It was a good time for us and we were ready.

We tried for several months. I believe we would have conceived sooner but neither of us was particularly good at math, so during April and May we tried during the wrong weeks. I had also been diagnosed with Polycystic Ovarian Syndrome, which affects an estimated 6 to 10 percent of women and is thought to be one of the leading causes of infertility. Its symptoms and their severity vary. In my case, my eggs were never released from my ovaries. I was fortunate that I was trying to conceive at thirty. As my gynecologist explained, being relatively young can help in treatment. After two low-dose cycles of the drug Clomid, along with a better understanding of the calendar, we witnessed the appearance of two pink lines on a plastic stick. We were pregnant.

That same day, the day I saw those pink lines, I bought several books on pregnancy. That night I read in horror about all the things that could go wrong. At least I could be prepared.

My next step was to take a prenatal class. There were prenatal yoga, prenatal workouts, natural birthing classes, and even a course on breast-feeding. In my third month I found a weekly prenatal workout class that met at six o'clock in the evening. The class focused on toning the transverse muscle, which is like a belt high in the abdomen under the breasts. I was told that if my transverse muscle was thoroughly toned, I would be able to literally push my baby out like toothpaste from a tube. Looking back, the class seemed a bit silly, but I had no point of reference back then. Both Peter and I felt compelled to participate in the grand preparation of childbirth.

The class also taught the pelvic floor exercises known as Kegels. Invented by Dr. Arnold Kegel in 1948, they are simple hold and

7

release repetitions meant to tone and strengthen the pubococcygeus muscle. As it was described to me, the pubococcygeus muscle is responsible for keeping you from peeing when you laugh or sneeze. By keeping the muscles in your pelvic floor toned you may not tear as much during labor or have a prolapsed uterus, and you would be more likely to manage the pain of labor.

The instructor reminded me of a camp counselor I once had at Acting Camp. She was all piss and vinegar, wore bright primary colors and large geometric earrings, which went well with her close-cropped salt-and-pepper hair. She explained, "Imagine yourself sitting on the floor cross-legged. Then pretend to pick up a penny using your vagina."

I understood the concept, but the idea of grabbing loose change with my vagina conjured up images of a weird sex show. However, Kegels could be done anywhere without detection. I Kegeled away on the subway, at the dinner table, and in meetings. I couldn't help but feel smug as I sat there strengthening my pubococcygeus muscle. I was preparing for childbirth while everyone else around the conference table was doing nothing.

Husbands attended only the orientation class and even though Peter had a pubococcygeus muscle, there was no need for him to strengthen his. Peter wanted to be more involved, so we signed up for a couples' class. It was a six-session course on natural childbirth. With the pain of labor months away, the drug-free natural birthing class was an easy choice.

Once a week at six-thirty we would take our seats on the floor and sit through three hours of instruction and films. I had been looking forward to the class, but getting up from the floor every half hour to pee soon made those Tuesday nights something I dreaded. Our fellow students were an eclectic mix. This being Manhattan, there was the token trendy young model couple, as well as several couples that looked to be ex-hippies in their mid-forties and two couples with heavy Eastern European accents. Most interesting was a woman who said her husband had several wives. She even brought a "sister wife" to class. There were also several show-offs, the type of people who would and did say, "I just finished reading several books on childbirth and what I found interesting is . . ." One woman would interrupt the instructor to add her own opinions.

The class watched instructional films on a small TV monitor. The natural home-birth film looked like it was shot on some commune in the seventies. There were a dozen fully dressed people standing around a grunting naked woman. The camera went in for an extreme close-up of her bloody vagina and the crown of a baby's head slipping through. When the film was over the instructor turned on the lights.

"Food break," she said.

In addition to the three-hundred-and-change tuition, we were all asked to bring in food for the break. Someone kept bringing in soft cheese, which is off-limits to the pregnant because it could harbor dangerous bacteria like *Listeria*. More suspicious perhaps were some of the homemade green and brown mystery dips. At the end of the third session we discovered our car had been towed. We took it as a sign, and didn't return to the class again. I had become preoccupied with other worries.

My triple-screen blood test had come back sketchy. I was just on the cusp of the statistical odds of our baby having an abnormality. My detailed sonogram had revealed other risk factors, which made an amniocentesis a necessity. I hyperventilated during the procedure and lost much of my early bravado. Peter and I decided not to engage in any "What if" conversations until we received the results. A few days later, our genetic counselor called us early in the morning with the good news. "I didn't want you to worry, we got the results of the amnio and they were all normal." In my heart of hearts I knew our baby would be okay. We knew it was a she. We peeked during the detailed sonogram. I believe the technician said something like, "I don't see a penis."

In my last few months of pregnancy I could barely get through my workday. The baby was seriously encroaching on my lungs, I was short of breath, and it seemed like everything gave me heartburn. I had cut back on my hours, but to get everything done I worked double time. The television series, with its thirteen episodes, was my first executive producing gig. There were producers, editors, and other staffers to deal with, not to mention all the notes and changes from the children's channel. I had three edit suites going at once and the last episode was to be delivered two weeks before my due date. I had never been as busy as I was during my pregnancy.

In my thirty-second week I was sitting in the office at my computer and felt pains from my abdomen. My midwife Suzanne told me to come downtown to her office. I was strapped onto a monitor. I was having contractions.

Before I knew it, I was hooked up to an IV at the hospital. They weren't sure what brought on the contractions. It could have been something I ate or the hours I put in at the office. Whatever the reason, the fluids I received intravenously were able to stop the contractions. I wasn't dilated and later that evening I was released. I was put on semi–bed rest from there on. What semi–bed rest meant to me was taking a car service to and from work.

Right around that time I began to retain fluid. I'm not sure if this happened because I was no longer able to take long walks and exercise or if it was inevitable. Either way I had a mild case of edema. Edema is the accumulation of fluids in the tissues, which if excessive causes swelling. It is very common in pregnancy and a mild case is considered normal. Not long after that, I was driven batty by the tingling and numbness I felt in both hands. I was told that the onset of carpal tunnel syndrome was common in pregnant women, usually brought on by hormonal changes and the accumulation of fluids. The good news—it was temporary and would most likely subside after delivery. Two over-the-counter ACE wrist supports brought some

10

relief and minimized the tingling. I wore them all the time, only taking them off to shower and use the ladies' room.

Fatigued and stressed, I never made it to the breast-feeding class. I remember thinking breast-feeding instruction was a waste of time. "It's the most natural thing in the world," I assured Peter when he asked if I should try and take the make-up. I was given my layette at my shower, and though a layette has nothing to do with nursing, in my mind I was ready. And we had hired a doula.

I had picked up a pamphlet on labor-support doulas at my prenatal workout class. The word *doula* is Greek meaning, "mothering the mother." We'd attended a doula workshop where we'd heard different birth stories along with statistics that showed the presence of a labor-support doula reduced rates of C-sections and epidurals. I was sold, especially when I met Maria. She was supportive, had a lovely accent from her native Venezuela, and had a toddler of her own. Empathetic by trade, her big smile made us feel at ease. I also liked the fact that when I did go into labor, Maria would come to our home and travel with us to the hospital. While Peter parked the car, I wouldn't have to be alone.

My original birthing plan was to stay at home as long as possible, breathing through the contractions. I had imagined the whole scenario. Just before transition, which is the third phase of labor when the final three centimeters of dilatation occurs, right before it's time to push, I would hop into a cab, go right to the delivery room, push, and presto, with no drugs I would be handed my baby. I wanted to be one of those women who had that special kind of plumbing where labor pains weren't that intense. I heard several stories about these women and later met a few. But I began to suspect I wasn't one of them. I was scared. My ankles were the same circumference as my thighs. I was open to drugs, and dreaded every day as I gained several pounds a week. Our new plan was to get to the hospital when I was in pain. It was that simple.

I couldn't wait to get through the hard part. Yes, I thought labor was the hard part. Tip number one: it isn't. I had been particularly labor focused for the last nine months and couldn't wait for the next phase, the mommy phase. I was exhausted and huge, bloated with forty-four pounds of baby, water, and pregnancy cravings. There were also certain expectations about my due date, which was coincidentally my husband's birthday, which was coincidentally his father's birthday. Now, the odds of our baby being born on the same day as her father and grandfather were 133,225 to one. So on Sunday night of April twenty-second, right after ten o'clock to be exact, I was relieved the games had begun. Three generations born on the same day would be my first great story.

And just how did the great event all begin? I ate spicy food and watched *Jackass*. I came upon this supposed labor inducer by chance. True, I had eaten extra-spicy Rigatoni FraDiavlo for dinner. Spicy food has long been suggested to bring on contractions. And I had taken calcium and evening primrose the whole week. The mineral/herb combination is purported to induce labor, too. But the exact moment that my labor began was when I turned on the show *Jackass*, gazed at my 23" TV screen, and saw a grown man dressed in a Santa suit receive a colonic. That was all it took. I heard a loud snap from somewhere within my pelvis. Labor was unmistakable.

I called Suzanne. "Try and get some sleep. At some point the contractions are going to wake you up," she instructed.

In bed, too excited to sleep, I thought back on the last nine months. Since the moment I understood that babies come out that tiny hole, I wondered, "How much pain?" Is it like the moment a needle is inserted for a shot, but for hours? Is it like a long menstrual cramp or the pain of an ingrown toenail? On my last visit with my midwife, the baby's weight had been estimated at nine pounds. What does it really feel like to have a nine-pound human come out of your vagina?

I woke at four-thirty in the morning and nudged Peter awake. The contractions felt like intense menstrual cramps. " I can do this," I told him, but I was really saying this for myself.

My pedicure, done in Bordeaux Red, had yet to chip. My manicure had that just-done shine. I had been getting manicures every other day for the last two weeks, reminding myself that you never know when you're going to go into labor. My legs were still smooth from a full leg wax. By the way, getting your legs waxed in your ninth month takes some contorting. You can't lie on your stomach for the back of the leg, so you lift and twist, but it was all worth it. I didn't want to look all messed up like those pictures people have of themselves right after they deliver a baby.

Now all I had to do was take a shower, blow-dry my newly layered cut, and put in my hot rollers. I would wear just some sheer foundation and lots of powder. I didn't want to look too overdone. An internal wrench, this time from my back muscles, stopped me in the shower. I just stood there as the pain wrapped around me. Once the pain reached the inside of my pelvis it would release. And then there would be nothing. I could manage this. This wasn't so bad. It was five in the morning on my due date, April twenty-third. Out of the shower, I called Suzanne again. She explained that I could expect to head to the hospital around noon.

"This is going to take a while," she assured me. About twenty minutes later we called her again.

"It's getting intense." Again she insisted that it would be a while. We called our labor support doula, Maria.

The labor pains, which were intermittent, were getting stronger. I found it impossible to curl my multi-layered hair. The complicated style was proving a wrong move. I was hoping to talk Maria into coming to our house sooner rather than later, but she, too, made me understand how long the process of labor could be.

Finally Maria arrived at six forty-five. She found me in our bedroom sitting in my combed cotton-maternity pajamas on my inflatable gym ball. The pajamas were an early purchase, which proved to be my favorite buy. When home I had worn nothing else.

"How will I know when I'm in active labor?" I asked Maria.

"We won't be able to carry on a conversation."

Suddenly I could no longer speak. Perhaps it was the power of suggestion or just that the right amount of time had passed. The bags were packed. My hair definitely didn't look the way I had hoped. I got up from the blue gymnastic ball, walked over to my closet, removed my pajamas, and put on a pair of black pants, my favorite cotton shirt from Liz Lange, and zipped up the sides of my Easy Spirit size-ten ankle boots. My size-nine shoes with their heels and designer labels were packed away somewhere next to my size-eight clothes.

Peter, Maria, and I headed down our three-flight walk-up. I couldn't breathe through the contractions, which were brought on with each step. Contractions made mind over matter impossible. The pain grew, reaching a crescendo and then slowly descended. So I felt the pain as it increased, and knew it was coming, that it would soon overtake me. I was thinking, "This is painful, oh this is more painful, no it just got even more painful, OK, I'VE HAD ENOUGH!" Then the grip loosened. And there I was in zero pain, a nice pause, and then I'd feel that twinge taking over.

Fifteen minutes later we were out by the car. My husband helped me go into the back seat. I don't have the most vivid memory of Peter other than him driving and being thrilled that our baby would share his and his father's birthday. Peter wondered if we would make the news. I couldn't really think about getting press at that moment. He said something like, "What a great birthday present." I hadn't bought Peter anything for his birthday. The baby would cover up that fact.

At nine sharp my husband dropped me off in front of the hospital and went to park the car. Maria and I inched our way through the lobby on my inflatable gym ball. I looked like I was riding a Hippity Hop in slow motion. My legs couldn't be trusted for walking. The contractions and the deep ache they brought made me double over. At least the ball provided some relief. The ball's forgiving surface let me move with the contraction, its surface giving way to my squirms and squats. I highly recommend getting the twenty-six-inch size. Many companies make them; mine was from Total Sports America. Toward the end of my pregnancy it had become my favorite place to sit. I even sat on it during my book group. Somehow I was moved to a wheelchair. The singular thought was on my mind: drugs. Any drugs, as long as they could take away the pain. Had someone offered me crack at that moment, I would have considered it. I wasn't "managing" any of it. I was desperate.

"We have to wait for your midwife to see if we can admit you. Then we can give you an epidural." The nurse was steadfast. The one thing they could start was my IV. The nurse noticed my wrist supports and we both agreed the IV should go in my left wrist because I was right-handed.

"See if Suzanne is anywhere on the floor," I told a flushed Peter, who joined us after parking the car.

"Isn't there anyone else here?" I asked the nurse. So much for loyalty in the grips of a contraction. Suzanne showed up minutes later. She examined me. I was four centimeters dilated and was admitted. I was able to get my epidural.

The attending anesthesiologist had me sit on the side of the bed, legs hanging off. I held the hands of the resident in front of me and the attending told me to make like a shrimp. I curved my back forward and bent my neck down as far as it would go. The hardest part was staying still. I felt the pressure of the needle, but it didn't hurt.

I was all business. I stayed completely still even during a contraction. After a few minutes, it was done.

I felt better . . . for about an hour. Hooked up to an IV, I watched bag after bag of liquid drip into me. I was bloating up even more. Then the contractions became painful again.

"I feel the pain again. Do you realize I am almost two hundred pounds? I think I need more pain medication." I didn't understand why I wasn't numb.

"You're ten centimeters." I had gone four centimeters to ten in an hour. Things were moving fast. I looked at Suzanne who was wearing one of those doctor space suits.

"What are you doing in those clothes?"

"You're ready to push. You think I'd be wearing these hot clothes if you weren't?" Suzanne took her seat in front of me.

"What? I just got my epidural, now I'm in pain again," I wondered aloud. Where was my down time? The monitor around my stomach signaled a contraction was coming. I knew pain was on its way before I felt the slightest twinge.

Penny, the nurse, picked up my smooth, hairless right leg. Maria grabbed the left. Suzanne was in the middle between them. I could see the deep red of my toenails peeking out. This was it. All those classes and exercises were going to be put to the test. My pelvic floor was in shape from all of my Kegels. I was ready to breathe out with my contractions, while using my toned transverse muscle to push.

"Okay, when you begin to feel the contraction, I want you to hold your breath and push like you're going to the bathroom!" Penny instructed. "Push like you're pooping," she reiterated. "You know how it feels when you have to go to the bathroom?"

What happened to pushing my baby out like toothpaste? Now we're down to poop? I suppose everything is a growth industry, but had someone just told me that we push our babies out like we are going to the bathroom I would have saved hundreds of dollars on all

16

those classes. Going to the bathroom—now that I can do. For the next two hours the words push and poop seemed pretty much the same. Somehow my waxed legs, pedicure, and manicure all lost their luster under those conditions.

Peter was a little too interested in the whole miracle of birth.

"Hey, don't look down there. What do you think this is, operating theater?" I hissed at him. "You think this is The Learning Channel?"

"Peter's doing a great job and I've seen it all," Penny offered.

"He's really been wonderful," Suzanne said.

"Most fathers usually aren't this interested," Maria added. Lucky for them I was all tied up. When I accused Peter of standing on my IV, Suzanne and the nurse came right to his defense once again. I was the one in pain doing all the work. But now it was Peter who was bonding with everyone.

When Peter wasn't transfixed down there, he remembered his one job, which consisted of putting a cool compress on my head.

No one can prepare you for the sounds of labor. But let me tell you, they are very similar to the sounds from a science-fiction movie like *Alien*, quick and slurpy.

A loud, wet, swishy noise would make me ask, "Is that the baby?"

"Nope," I was told. And I would lie there thinking, "Well, what was it?" Each push produced another one for the sound library. You know when you watch the Oscars and they have that segment on sound effects? They show a scene with laser beams batting back and forth. And then they cut to some guy in a studio recording the sound of wet dog food sliding out of a can. And everyone in the audience is wowed thinking who knew it was dog food making that laser sound. In fact, all one really needs to do is record the sounds of birth.

"One more time, just like before," the nurse instructed. "Oh, you're so good at this. Other women don't get it like you do and remember, push like you're going to the bathroom." My nurse said this all in one breath. I thought to myself, I'm good at this.

There is also a lot of false praise in that little room. My husband would later tell me that I was nowhere with the pushing, but they just lied and lied. "Oh she's almost here. One more." They even asked me if I wanted a mirror. Not only did I not want to look down there, I had no intention of ever looking down there again. Then there was that one moment when it hurt more than anything in the world, when it felt like a burn and pull all at once. My husband was silent.

Later he told me, "It should have hurt. Her head was halfway out." I pushed again.

"Push, push." And I pushed and pushed. Of course we all knew at this point what they meant by "pushing." "Stop, stop, oh, push push."

"She has lots of black hair!" Penny our nurse told me. Finally, after nearly an hour and a half of pushing, it was perfectly clear to me how to get our baby out.

"Pull it! Pull it!" I screamed. If they simply grabbed some of that black hair and gave a good yank we'd all be done.

"Oh no, it's up to you, Mommy. Come on, give a push, ready, push push." The nurse cheered me on.

"Stop, stop, push, push," my midwife yelled.

And with one giant thrust, our daughter, Sophie, came into the world at two twenty-three in the afternoon. Suzanne placed our little girl on my chest. I was starstruck.

"Here she is," Peter said as he stroked the back of her head. There was nothing I could say. Peter kissed me.

"Can you believe it? She arrived right on time. This was her due date," Peter told the room. "She's the third generation born on April twenty-third. It's my dad's birthday, my birthday, and now her birthday."

"Happy birthday, Peter," Suzanne said.

"Happy birthday, what a great present," the nurse told Peter. It was a coincidence, a happy one, but I needed the attention. If I wasn't on so many drugs I might have said something like, "Don't mind me, why don't you all go out and celebrate." But I couldn't really put a sentence together, much less a sarcastic one. Maybe it was the drugs, but I was loopy and wanted the little baby cleaned up. I couldn't help but think that it was my gooey stuff covering her from head to toe. She had finally arrived.

That's that, I thought. The hard part was over.

Chapter 2

Don't Bite Your Newborn

WE HAD A HEALTHY baby girl, seven pounds, thirteen ounces, nineteen and a half inches long. She wasn't the predicted nine pounds, which was a relief. Sophie scored 9 on her Apgar test. Her head was perfectly round and now that she had been bathed we saw she had beautiful black curly hair.

"I'm done." Tanked up on Percocet, I asked, "Are there any other drugs?"

"Demerol."

"OK, give me Demerol." There it was, another pill.

"You have to push." Suzanne was firm.

"Push? I already pushed the baby out."

No one was going to get me to do anything. I was relaxing now. My husband was holding our gorgeous baby. I was stunned. I had just given birth. I was trying to decide which hurt more, the contractions or pushing. It was a tie.

"You need to push out the placenta," Suzanne insisted.

"Just pull it out. You have the cord." Peter had done the honors and cut the umbilical cord, so I knew they had the cord. I had lost all sense of time, how many minutes, how many hours. Of course I wanted to get the placenta out, but I just didn't have the presence of mind to understand that I needed to work at it. Pushing was hard and I was holding back for fear of more pain.

Finally, after what Peter told me was forty minutes, Suzanne said softly in my ear, "You better push or I'm sending you to the OR." This was a complication. I wasn't done, and I needed to get with it. I held my breath and pushed real hard.

"Is that the placenta?" Peter asked. "It's huge."

"The placenta is the body's only disposable organ," Suzanne informed us. It looked like a giant liver.

With Maria there, Peter finally asked if he could take a break. Next he did what any all-American new dad would do after watching the afterbirth come out of his wife. He left the hospital, walked two blocks uptown to the closest McDonalds, and wolfed down a double cheeseburger value meal, supersized.

Meanwhile, I tried not to look down as Suzanne sewed up my tear.

"Is it bad?" I didn't really want to know the answer.

"No, it's not that big. It just went through several folds. . . ." I zoned out as she answered my question in far more detail than I'd hoped. I stared at Sophie instead, occasionally catching a glimpse of Suzanne pulling the thread and needle through. An hour ago Sophie was still inside me, now she was a perfect little creature there in her bassinet.

Finally Suzanne was done. She stood up and in an authoritative tone said, "Now no sex for six weeks. Okay?"

I couldn't believe Suzanne actually had to tell me that, after having cross-stitched a sampler down there.

I was given a new hospital gown and was asked if I could move my legs, which I could. Somehow I got out of bed and into a wheelchair.

"We have a private room, right?" I asked.

"That's where I'm taking you." Penny pushed my wheelchair down the hall and into our private room. Then she rushed out and returned with the rest of my belongings.

"I want to say good-bye and thank you," I told her.

"Oh, I'll be right back." Penny said it like she was going to come back. I waited, thinking we would hug. I just assumed that's what our delivery nurse and I would do. Maybe we'd snap off a few photos. We were close now, bonded by the event of my daughter's birth.

We never saw her again. Looking back I am not sure why I noticed this. I guess I wanted a proper good-bye from the lady who an hour or so before coached me through labor with her favorite cheer, "Push like you're pooping."

A NEW NURSE came in wearing a loud, colorful print. If you're going to wear scrubs with grinning pandas all over it, the least you can do is crack a smile, but there was no, "Welcome, congratulations on your new baby. How wonderful, my name is so-and-so and if you need anything just buzz."

Instead it went something like, "Let me know when you want to use the bathroom." She wrote something down on her clipboard and walked out. The distance from the delivery room to my recovery room was the length of two short hallways, but it felt like a great chasm. The attention paid to me as an expectant mother was gone. Now I was a first-time mom, which seemed like a totally different class: a lower class.

The room was sterile and had the same lighting as an airplane bathroom, the kind that beckons you into an impromptu facial. It smelled of witch hazel, but it had a wonderful view of Greenwich Village and downtown Manhattan, and I was relieved to find I had my own bathroom and shower. The hospital encouraged rooming in with the baby instead of taking the newborn to the nursery. So there was a baby in the room.

That baby was mine.

She was safe in her bassinet nearly asleep, but I had Peter hand her to me just so I could hold her. "I can't believe we have a baby." I would say that several times that night and likewise Peter kept saying it to me. I really couldn't grasp it. She looked stylish in her newborn nightie and matching hat, both gifts from my shower.

Maria came to my bedside to ask if I was ready to nurse. I wasn't. Though I envisioned tender mommy moments of myself nursing my baby, the actual act of bringing the baby to my breast was something I hadn't contemplated.

"Thank you so much, you don't have to stay. I'll have one of the nurses help me." Still hooked up to the IV and several other tubes, I hugged Maria, or at least mimed a hug good-bye.

Maria left, but I was far from alone. Family began to trickle in. My mother-in-law, Nola, was glowing. "Her head's not misshapen at all." She rubbed Sophie's soft hairy head many times that evening.

My father-in-law, Harry, kept saying, "Another miracle." The big conversation, aside from how lovely and perfect Sophie was, focused on the happy coincidence of shared birthdays. My parents, Mike and Lucy, arrived soon after. My mom kept wiping her eyes. When my older sister Anne arrived she grew teary eyed as well.

This was the first grandchild on both sides and everyone looked dazed. I guess I was too. I had yet to cry over the baby. I was happy, but mostly amazed. My one friend with children told me she cried both times she brought her babies home, right when she walked through the front door. I figured that was when I would cry.

When you have a baby, everyone, even the sister you've been feuding with for the last decade shows up a card-carrying aunt. All bets and grudges are off. Everyone is genuinely elated. I had seen my younger sister Edith only once in the last year, at my baby shower.

Now she was snapping away picture after picture. Perhaps it's because they'd never seen me look so bad or it's because I was holding their new niece in my arms. Sophie's eyes looked fused shut and she didn't seem to mind the flash. Peter kept leaning in over the bed to get in the shot. Those photos made their way into the baby book. Even though I looked all moon-faced and greasy, they were our first family photos.

The hospital's version of dinner arrived. Aside from the chocolate pudding, nothing looked particularly edible. Perhaps it was the presentation, all Styrofoam and plastic wrap. But it had been nearly twenty hours since I last ate. I was hungry. Tea and Sympathy, a cozy English tea shop located three blocks from the hospital, has the best macaroni and cheese in the city. They also have wonderful Welsh rarebit, Victorian sandwich, and shepherd's pie, but that first day of motherhood I was craving a childhood favorite. And though I've been told many times that having ketchup mixed in with macaroni and cheese is gross, there is no better way as far as I'm concerned. Peter called in the order and ran out to pick it up.

I didn't think twice about eating a big fattening meal. I was in desperate need of a treat and I knew that nursing burns an additional 500 calories a day. That's 200 more than the 300 extra calories a day I required when I was pregnant. For the last three weeks I had been on a strict no sweet/no carbohydrate diet to control my rapid weight gain, which wasn't entirely due to edema. I indulged that last trimester and paid for it. And so now with Sophie safely delivered, my food fantasies took on an almost pornolike quality. I daydreamed about the pastel frostings of Magnolia Bakery's fifties-style cupcakes. I longed for the milk chocolate peanut butter crisps from Bon Bons, the Long Island chocolatier, or milk chocolates from See's Candies. I wanted almond croissants from Jon Vie for breakfast, creamy macaroni and cheese for lunch, and a dinner of fried chicken and biscuits. All of this would be supplemented with chocolate malts and spoonfuls of Nutella right out of the jar. And what would happen to me with all this forbidden food? I would shrink back down to a size eight in a matter of weeks, nursing away all those calories. It seems fitting that the very first home movies that Peter took of Sophie have her asleep in her Plexiglas bassinet and me a fuzzy figure in the background, stuffing my face. Not quite the image found in those mommy and baby commercials.

The truth was maybe I was distracting myself from the task at hand. I was nervous about putting Sophie to my breast. There was no escaping it; soon the nurse would return and I would need to latch my baby on. A latch, for the uninitiated, is the point of contact between a baby's mouth and a mother's breast while nursing. While I was pregnant, the baby was a fantasy. She existed in my daydreams where I controlled what happened and how I looked. When I imagined myself nursing I was usually humming a lullaby while rocking back and forth in my new glider.

I had told our delivery nurse that I planned to breast-feed. On Sophie's pink ID card, which was taped to the side of her bassinet, the word "breast" was written in the upper right-hand corner like a contract.

Medical science has proven in study after study the benefits of nursing. I had enough knowledge to know that I really didn't have a choice. My mother nursed me for six months and so far I've lived a healthy existence, fortunate to avoid chronic disease and allergies. Peter was also breast-fed, which may have accounted for his support. Though I hadn't taken the time to read up on how to nurse, I was obsessed with the statistics and findings about the benefits of nursing. Barring some physical obstacle, my breasts would be Sophie's source of nutrition.

I could have asked my mother or mother-in-law about nursing, but I was too self-conscious. I preferred dealing with a stranger.

With all our visitors saying their good-byes, I finally had enough privacy to try to pee. I pushed the red button next to my bed. About ten minutes later a nurse strolled in wearing scrubs with a dancing bunny print.

"Are you ready to try to eliminate?" the nurse asked.

"Do you think this is going to hurt?"

"I'm not going to lie, sometimes it does."

I got up from my bed and shuffled into the bathroom. The nurse rolled my IV behind me—it wouldn't be disconnected until I was successful. The nurse stood guard outside the door. For the first time since I delivered Sophie I was alone. In the mirror above the sink I saw an image I did not recognize. Comic in size, my face had been replaced by water-balloon cheeks and jowl. I knew my face had been puffy for the last few months, but what I saw made me sad. I didn't look like the glowing new mom I pictured. Instead I was swollen beyond recognition. I wished I knew where I had put my lipstick. I wanted to do something. Embarrassed by my appearance, I didn't want any more hospital visitors or photos.

"How's it going in there?" the nurse asked, reminding me of my original mission.

Though I feared I would feel excruciating pain, the act of peeing was surprisingly pain-free.

"It went all right. I'm done," I called back.

The nurse came in holding a giant maxi pad.

"You're going to need this." She bent the maxi in half and shook it vigorously. I was confused, and briefly wondered if I was seeing things through my Percocet/Demerol haze. That is, until she handed me the ice-cold maxi pad. It had an ice pack inside it, which had been activated by all her shaking.

There are two things a new mom should hoard while at the hospital. The first item is that ice-pack maxi pad. Remember they aren't cold unless you bend and shake them. Be sure to ask for it right after delivery and change them often. I'm convinced I didn't have swelling because of those ice pads. Ask different nurses for supplies, being

26

careful not to ask the same nurse twice. Once they're on to you, it will be nearly impossible to stock up. You'll hit your best payload right after shift changes.

The second must-haves are disposable panties. Made of a white form-fitting mesh material, they are much more comfortable than regular briefs. You just toss them in the trash once they get dirty. And they will get dirty. You'll need them for your first week home because after you've had a baby you are going to bleed, and that first week you may bleed like you are having the heaviest period in the world. So those disposable panties are a must. They are difficult to track down in stores and can be relatively expensive, so take my advice and stash what you can.

Once I was back in bed, the nurse unhooked my IV.

"I'd like to try and nurse her now." It had been about an hour and a half since I delivered Sophie. Peter was sitting next to me on the bed.

The only breast-feeding information I had with me was contained in a slim pamphlet on nursing published by some formula company. I actually loved the way it tucked nicely in my weekend bag's side pocket. The cover had a picture of a woman in a turtleneck sitting in a rocker with a small baby ever so delicately sucking from her breast. That was my image of nursing.

"I need help latching her on." This was the extent of my nursing terminology. I pulled out my breast.

The nurse took one look at my nipple and said, "You need to bring the nipple out." The nurse bent forward. There she was in my business, squeezing my nipple. I wasn't ready for that. It's true my nipples were usually flat by day, but weren't everyone's? They always seemed to perk up when they needed to.

"What do you mean?" I asked. There I was, thirty-one years old, just finding out that my nipples aren't "out."

"Just bring it out, Mommy." The nurse pinched my breast. She was the second person to call me by my new name, Mommy.

Mommy was how most of the hospital staff addressed new moms. At first it was a novelty, but later when I had a better ear for the nurses' patronizing tone, "mommy" sounded a lot like "dummy." The nurse pinched my breast again. My flat nipples and the problems they can cause didn't really sink in for days. In denial I thought, "Bring the nipple out" was some sort of breast-feeding pre-latch cheer. "Bring it out, yeah team!"

I remembered seeing plastic breast shells at Buy Buy Baby, which read "For flat or inverted nipples." I walked by thinking, "Glad that's not me." But it was.

Then there was little Sophie. The nurse helped me bring her to my breast. Sophie flailed about, her mouth open and eager, her head turning every which way with unsavory snorts and cries coming from her tiny mouth. The nurse took my arm and placed Sophie in it. Her head was in my hand and her legs straddled my arm. Holding both my hand and Sophie's head the nurse pushed Sophie directly into my breast.

Sophie looked like she was latched onto my breast, but those pictograph's in the pamphlet weren't the best point of reference. More confusing was the silence. Her mouth was moving, but it didn't sound like she was getting anything. There wasn't a gulp. There wasn't a swallow.

"Oh, they get something," the nurse said as she left the room. I doubted this, but I was so unsure myself that I chalked it up to being a rookie. The total amount of time the nurse spent with me was about three minutes.

I tried to picture my little nursling getting milk or more accurately, the colostrum. Colostrum is an extremely nutritious dense yellow liquid, rich in antibodies, that comes in before one's milk. I read in my pamphlet that it was all a baby needs in the beginning. I nursed her, or thought I nursed her, two more times that night.

Since we had a private room, Peter spent his first night as a new dad in the other hospital bed. Had there been more deliveries that afternoon we might not have been so lucky.

The next day Sophie fell asleep every time I brought her to my breast. She was excited as I brought her in, crying and making little piggy sounds. Then once she was on or what I thought was a latch she would fall asleep and not even attempt to nurse.

By the afternoon it was clear why Sophie was so groggy. She was jaundiced. Her body wasn't able to process and eliminate her bilirubin, a pigment produced by the normal breakdown of oxygen-carrying red blood cells. Her bilirubin count was climbing, and if left unchecked severe jaundice can damage brain cells. Peter and I had an ABO blood incompatibility, which caused Sophie's jaundice. I had made antibodies to Sophie's blood type, which was the same as my husband's. To add to this, Sophie's cord blood had been misplaced sometime after delivery. I saw Suzanne take the blood. She labeled the tubes and everything, but for whatever reason they never made it to the lab. Later, when it was discovered the cord blood had been lost, one of the residents urged us to lodge an official complaint. Maybe we should have, but we only thought of Sophie that afternoon. It wasn't that we were ambivalent. We were upset, especially since Sophie required additional heel sticks. But it was too much for us to process.

A young female pediatric resident was the first to tell me she thought Sophie was looking yellow. It had happened so gradually I hadn't noticed how olive yellow she had become. A blood incompatibility can be serious. At one point the staff had discussed a blood transfusion.

Right after the resident gave me the results of her blood test, the pediatrician called. He had the delivery of a Borscht Belt veteran, "Mommy, this is what we're going to do. We're going to put her in sunglasses. She's going to look like she's ready for Miami. We're going to place her under the lights. The lights are going to break down the bilirubin. And you're going to need to pump. See, to get the bilirubin out, we're going to give her lots of liquids. So we're going to cupfeed her formula and whatever milk you're able to pump. Now, the cup is neutral so it won't interfere with breastfeeding. She's going to have explosive bowel movements and your breasts are going to feel like Rocks of Gibraltar. Ask the nurse for a breast pump. Every three hours you can take her out to nurse, but you're not going to be able to have her too long. That's why she'll also need the formula and, like I said, you'll need to pump. She's going to be fine. They wanted to put her in the NICU (Neonatal Intensive Care Unit) but instead they're going to move the phototherapy crib into your room, so she'll be with you. This should clear up in the next day or so."

I didn't know how to respond. I was happy that she would be staying with us in our room, but I worried that they would release me before Sophie. I couldn't watch another heel stick. There had been several that afternoon and each time the nurse pricked her heel, she would cry, she was in pain, and I felt helpless.

Soon after I hung up with the doctor a nurse came in with a cylinder bottle of formula and a tiny shot-size plastic cup. The nurse got right to work. She crossed her legs and nestled Sophie between her thigh and bent leg. When I held Sophie she seemed so fragile, but the way this nurse handled her Sophie seemed sturdy and strong. The nurse was able to prop Sophie up into a sitting position and put a cloth diaper under her chin, like a bib. Then she filled the cup halfway with formula, brought it to Sophie's lips, and tilted it into her mouth. Sophie took gulps. The way Sophie sat there she looked like a tiny robot swallowing each time she was offered a drink. "See how they can drink out of a cup?" The nurse smiled at me. The nurse kept pouring more formula into the tiny cup. Sophie took several ounces. When Sophie refused to take another sip, the nurse handed her back to me. "That's how you'll cupfeed her."

The pediatric resident came in pushing a giant criblike device into our room. She and the nurse maneuvered the contraption next to my bed. The nurse left and the resident took Sophie, stripped her down to her diaper, placed a protective eye cover on Sophie's face, turned on the crib's blue lights, pulled down the Plexiglas side, and placed Sophie inside the infant tanning bed. "This should clear it out." And with that the resident left the room. Peter and I could do nothing but stare at our little blue Sophie.

I PUSHED that red button again. The nurses had changed shifts, and a new evening nurse came in. She was dressed in a white classic nurse's uniform complete with skirt. She was older and seemed confused when I requested a breast pump. I hadn't expected to cross that bridge for a few months. I assumed that pumping was something I would do later on, when I went back to work.

The nurse returned with a small sterile package that read, "Manual Breast Pump." She opened the package and looked at its contents as though she herself had never seen a breast pump before. It was a plastic yellow-and-white contraption that contained a metal spring about four inches long. It had a clear bottle and a funnel not unlike the one I used for baking at home. The nurse looked over the instructions for several minutes, and then handed them to me along with the package. Without a word she left the room. Peter and I were dumbfounded. It was bizarre, but true. The nurse couldn't be bothered with helping us assemble the manual pump. She seemed so out of it, I didn't want to call her back. Instead Peter and I put it together.

After I was done screwing all the parts in place, I held in my hand what looked like one of those pumps I used to fill my bicycle tires with air.

"Do you think this is how it's supposed to go?" I asked Peter.

I handed him the pump and he looked it over trying to decide which end was up. "I have no idea." He handed it back to me. I put the pump's funnel to my breast. And with Peter sitting next to me, I compressed the handle.

Peter was constantly asking me if I needed anything. He was the one who asked the nurses for those ice maxi pads and mesh underwear. He brought me flowers that first morning in the hospital. Aside from errands, Peter did not leave my side, and since my in-laws took Halley for a few weeks, Peter didn't go home, not even for a change of clothes. And he was behind my breast-feeding one hundred percent. Even that plastic device didn't sway him. But we hadn't addressed our pumping etiquette. I hadn't decided if I was going to be the kind of wife who pumped in front of her husband, or the kind who locked the door. Though I think I was partial to the locked door. Likewise I don't think Peter was sure he wanted to be in the room. As supportive as Peter was with breast-feeding, he later admitted that he didn't know until that day that you could pump your breasts or needed to. But he didn't let on there in the hospital and rubbed my back while I pumped.

It was awkward and stressful, like the time our dog walker saw me naked.

As I compressed the handle, it felt like I was trying to pump my breast full of air. It was the same motion as an air pump. All of this was made more frustrating by the weak use of my hands. It was too early to tell if my wrists and hands would recover from the carpal tunnel, as far as I could tell they still ached. But still I pumped away. Nothing came out. My wrists hurt and I decided to try again later.

My breasts began to creep me out in general. They were heavy and had all these hard spots. They were something different, something uncomfortable. They were something alive.

When my mother visited for a second time I asked her about my breasts.

"I think they're supposed to get hard," my mom said, staring at Sophie who basked in the blue light of the phototherapy cage. Remembering a proper latch or how breasts are supposed to feel right after you give birth was something she said she just didn't recall. It had been twenty-eight years since she weaned my younger sister Edith. At this point my mom was happiest when she could find her car keys.

"You'll figure it out, it's natural." There was that word, natural. Natural was a brand name in my mind, it meant healthy. In terms of nursing, natural meant something I was instinctively supposed to know.

Another nurse came in to check on me.

"Could I show you something?" I called her close to my bed and lifted back both panels of my nursing bra, not the easiest thing to do with strangers, and whispered, "Does this look right to you?" The woman stepped back. She looked startled and her face turned a light crimson.

Backing out of the room she said, "I just came in to see if you wanted to do the rental for the TV and phone. I'll get a nurse to help you with your problem."

I couldn't believe I had just flashed the hospital's television-rental girl.

When the nurse came in I went through the whole show again.

"Oh, Mommy, your milk is coming in." The nurse checked Sophie and her light box and left the room. This was pretty much how the day went. I would alert the staff that my breasts felt hard and they would tell me that my milk was coming in. Every three hours I would ask to take Sophie out of her light box. We would pour formula down her throat using a little tiny cup. I would attempt to latch her on, eat macaroni and cheese and chocolate, and pump. During all of my attempts to nurse her, I never heard a gulp or swallow.

33

I kept trying to latch Sophie on, but it was like threading a needle on a bus. Intuitively I would gingerly bring her straight onto my breast, but she moved about wildly, growing more frantic the closer she came to me. The nurse would come back after about twenty minutes to cupfeed her supplemental formula. When she wouldn't drink another gulp it was time to place her back under the photo lights. I would try to pump, though I still was unable to get a single drop.

The next morning, a senior nurse came in. No loud prints with dancing pandas for her. Her dress was pure hospital scrub. She was upset to find a manual pump next to my bed. Disgusted, she left the room. Five minutes later she returned wheeling in the hospital-grade Medela Classic Breast Pump. It looked and sounded like a prop from the Mel Brooks movie *Young Frankenstein*. Because it was covered in clear plastic you could actually see how the machine worked. There was a motor thing moving some kind of piston thing, which moved some other kind of machine thing. It was an intimidating piece of equipment. Not only could it pump your breasts, but looked like it could rotate chicken. The nurse attached two long clear tubes to the machine. Then she attached two plastic funnels, which were connected to two plastic bottles. She asked me to double pump, but I made up my mind that I was a one-at-a-time kind of girl. The nurse tried to explain that I would get more milk if I double pumped but I just wasn't ready. It would be weeks before I understood physiologically that you get more milk double pumping. I brought the clear plastic funnel up to my breast and turned on the machine to its lowest setting. The machine made a rhythmic hiss and pucker.

HERE YOU ARE with your breasts, they've taken you through puberty, worked well for you all through college with a variety of boyfriends.

34

They were a nice round 36 B. And then there you are pumping. The very act of pumping one's breast is so completely alien, so unnatural, and yet the body responds. First I pumped the left breast, and then I pumped the right. I wasn't getting a great deal out of either breast, but a little began to trickle into the bottle. I should have had the electric pump right from the start. My advice for any new mom is never use a hand pump right after delivery. It just doesn't have the power and gentler settings you'll need. Demand a hospital-grade electric pump.

I had lost a lot of blood from the complication with my placenta and was approved to stay for an additional day, which brought me great relief. I had feared returning home to Brooklyn without our baby. Instead of being sent home the following morning we would spend the next day and night at the hospital. I knew I was lucky to have Peter with me, but in so many ways between pumping and nursing, I felt very much alone. I couldn't snuggle with my new daughter because she needed to be under the lights. When Peter hugged me I didn't want him to hold me tight, my chest was too tender. And I chose to pump when he ran errands. I was waiting for Sophie's bilirubin count to come down, for my milk to come in, and for me to feel that warm glow of new motherhood.

It must have been two or three in the morning on our second night in the hospital. The night nurse, the same one who gave me the hand pump, woke me. It was time to feed Sophie. Peter, still fully dressed in the clothes he'd worn to the hospital that first day, was half asleep in his bed. I sat down in one of the room's metal institutional chairs. The nurse handed Sophie to me and left the room. Sophie seemed tightly swaddled but she flailed about crying, shaking loose most of the blanket. Her little arms would cover her face and get in the way of the latch. I needed a third arm just to get her in position. At first I asked Peter to hold down her arms, but his hands got in the way. I knew if I could just move her tiny arm out of the way, I could get a good latch. Because I'm five foot nine, the distance from my newborn to my breast was nearly a foot. I hunched over, but the process wasn't working.

I wanted to be one of those problem-solving mothers. After all, I am a problem-solver. I was scared of heights yet I managed to climb Mt. Khatadin, the highest point in Maine. It took me two days and several Boy Scouts were forced to literally climb over me, but I did it. As a documentary filmmaker I had survived the world of women's boxing with its promoters and trainers and navigated the treacherous waters of New York's swing dance community. I was sure I could figure out how to nurse a baby.

I thought that if I picked up her arm by grabbing the sleeve of her shirt between my teeth I would be able to move Sophie into nursing position. I simply nabbed a little bit of cloth and was then able to pick up her arm. There she was, in position.

Sophie's mouth opened as far as it could go. At first she was silent. Then a scream, like nothing I have ever heard, came out of little Sophie.

"What happened?" Peter got out of bed. "What did you do?" I lifted back the sleeve of her shirt and spotted a confetti-sized bright red mark. I had just bitten my two day-old daughter.

"I think I bit her." A rush of guilt came over me. Were they going to take her away? I didn't do it on purpose.

"What? You bit her? How did you bite her?" My husband was upset. Sophie was crying. It hurt and she didn't know what was happening.

"I meant to pick up her arm, see." I showed him how it happened. "You think I did this on purpose?" I also immediately wanted to cover it up. In my two-day postpartum messed up state I was afraid they would take the baby. "Look I'll get the pediatrician to look at it. I'll say she got pinched by accident." I pressed the nurse button.

"Why would you try and move a baby's arm using your teeth?" Peter hovered over me.

36

"I told you, I went to pick up her shirt. See the fold in the cloth . . ." I tried again to explain. The nurse came in.

"I think I accidentally pinched our baby's arm." I explained to the nurse. I cried.

"Oh, that's not so bad." The nurse rubbed in some antibiotic cream. She told me that this wouldn't be the last time I would hurt our baby by accident.

That was it, ammunition for a lifetime. Whenever I'd say, "How did she fall off her bike? Weren't you watching her?"

"At least I didn't bite her," Peter could say.

"I'm taking Sophie to the park," I'd tell Peter.

"Try not to bite her honey, okay," Peter could call back.

"I told you, no fast food," I'd insist.

"At least I didn't bite her."

No sane person would accidentally bite her baby. Later I asked the pediatrician to look at her little arm with its bright red hole, where two teeth had met. I explained I accidentally pinched her, which in hindsight doesn't seem that much better than biting. It didn't faze him. And back she went under the lights.

My breasts were getting even harder. I had read in the hospital's Postpartum Discharge Instructions about engorgement and it developed into my worst fear.

"Your milk is just coming in," the nurse assured me. Then, about four hours later she changed her mind, "I think you're getting engorged."

"I've been telling you all I was feeling full and hard, now you tell me I'm engorged." I needed help. I needed to get out of the hospital.

Later that evening, Sophie's bilirubin count finally came down. Suzanne, our midwife, also came by to check on me. She asked how nursing was going. When I pulled back the panels of my nursing bra she immediately said, "They're red and irritated." Suzanne left the room and came back with two plastic doll-sized versions of goalie masks, like the ones Jason wears in those *Friday the Thirteenth* movies. Suzanne told me to wear them over my nipples. The shells are designed to keep clothing away from irritated skin. I took the shells and put them in place.

Suzanne suggested that we set up an appointment with a lactation consultant. Lactation consultants are certified health-care professionals who are experts in solving nursing-related problems. Through my various prenatal classes I had collected several pages of phone numbers and addresses of maternity shops, baby nurses, diaper supplies. In the mix there were also a few numbers for lactation consultants. It had never occurred to me that I would need one. Peter worked the phones. Though he mostly spoke with machines, he managed to get an appointment for Friday afternoon, a day and a half away. Sophie was nursing every two to three hours.

The next morning we got the good news. Sophie's bilirubin count continued to decrease. We could all go home. The bad news was my breasts were a mess. The morning nurse came into my room. She looked at me, or more specifically my breasts, and said, "You're really engorged."

You're officially engorged when you are producing more milk than you are expressing either through nursing or pumping. I was frightened. I was frightened that they could get bigger and harder. I was frightened of getting the breast infection, known as mastitis, which I read about in my little pamphlet.

BECAUSE SOPHIE was the first baby in the family, I was enjoying a new dynamic with both my sisters. They were single and let me know they were available for their new aunt duties. My older sister, Anne, had casually offered to help us get the baby home.

I called her early on Thursday and she arrived around ten in the morning. "So how long do you think you need me?" Anne seemed anxious.

"You said you would help." I was incredulous.

"I mean you won't be needing me the whole day?" Anne didn't bother to remove her coat. My sister worked on Wall Street and took pride in the fact that she no longer had to deal with the "end user." She had little patience for nurses or hospital bureaucracy.

"I don't know. I've never taken a baby home before." The nurse came in and handed me a clipboard with several documents on it.

"It's just I told the office I was stepping out for coffee." Anne added.

"Is that it?" I said to the nurse. I signed my signature several times without even reading the paperwork. I just wanted to get home. "Anne, I don't know how long, why didn't you tell your office you were helping your sister take your new niece home?"

"Didn't want to take a personal day." Anne sat down.

"That's it." The nurse handed me a large plastic diaper bag full of formula and coupons for more formula.

"We've been using the cup because I'm breast-feeding. Could I get a couple of those tiny cups?" She dashed out of the room for a brief moment and returned with a bag of tiny medicine cups. The nurse left the room again and return with a fist full of those tiny nipples that are designed to fit the small cylinder-like formula bottles used in hospitals. She tossed them into the diaper bag. "You might need these."

I felt defensive and paranoid all at once. I didn't like her implication that there was going to be a plan B. Defiant, I wanted to take the nipples out of the bag, but I couldn't. Did the nurse know I wasn't going to make it? Could they tell just by looking at me? Were the nurses placing bets on me? "Oh that big puffy one with the flat nipples thinks she's going to nurse. I bet she lasts two days." I would keep the nipples in the bag, but under no circumstances were we ever going to use them.

The nurse took the clipboard, checked my wrist ID as well as Sophie's, and cross-referenced it with the numbers on our paperwork. "Let me know when you're ready to go downstairs." With that the nurse walked out into the hall.

THE PLAN was simple. Peter and Anne would get our Corolla and install the infant car seat, which had become an issue between Peter and me. I had been nudging him to install it for the last two weeks.

"It'll take me five minutes," he told me several times. Keep in mind it took Peter and his father an entire day to assemble the crib. And there was also the time Peter took our new stroller out of the box and inadvertently tore off a wheel. But I decided against bringing up either incident.

While they went to get the car, I would dress the baby and bring her down to the lobby. We would pop by the drugstore, pick up a breast pump, and head to Brooklyn. I estimated that we would need my sister for about two hours.

Peter and Anne headed for the car. Alone in the hospital room it was time to dress my tiny baby. Though it's normal for babies to lose weight in the hospital, Sophie hadn't because the nurses had cupfed her formula to clear out the jaundice. But she was still yellow. I put Sophie in her going home outfit, which my mom had given us. With Sophie in her first civilian clothes, an oversized jacket and pant set, we were ready.

I took one more look at our hospital room. It's funny how one can get used to such a sterile setting. But with its panoramic view of the city and the sunlight streaming in it seemed less cold and foreign than it had the last few days. Perhaps that's because I was leaving. As I went to get the nurse I plucked Sophie's pink ID card from her Plexiglas bassinet. It would make a nice memento in her baby book.

40

I stared for a moment at that word written in the upper right corner, "breast."

I held Sophie in my arms as the nurse wheeled us down to the lobby. The nurse said goodbye and sped off back to the elevator. I wanted to yell back "I'm going to make it breast-feeding! You'll see. I don't need your nipples!" But I thought better of it. Instead I took a seat on a couch in the hospital's main lobby.

It had been forty-five minutes since Anne and Peter headed down to the car. Anne finally came in to get me.

"We're doubled parked across the street. Peter seems to be having some trouble," Anne told me on the QT. Peter was in an all out struggle with the car seat and our old Corolla. Sophie was asleep. If Sophie woke up, she would want to eat. I wouldn't have been able to breast-feed her in the car and I didn't know how we would manage to cupfeed her in the backseat. Finally the car seat was in place.

"Do you need me to go to the drugstore?" Anne dialed her voicemail again. We could hear the automated response through her cell phone, "No new messages."

"I've got a lot of big deals out there, I just don't want to miss a call," she said clutching her cell phone. "I've been so busy lately."

I explained to Anne that Peter had to get the pump, and that if we needed to move the car I didn't think I could do it. I really needed her to stay. We had reserved the pump at Bigelow's Pharmacy in the Village. I insisted on the same one we used at the hospital, the Medela Classic. The rental rate was two dollars a day. There are cheaper models to buy, but by renting I felt I could do away with performance anxiety.

The drugstore added another hour to our trip. As we drove home to Brooklyn I saw all the pink cherry blossoms, which were at their peak. Everyone in the city seemed to be playing hooky. It was the kind of weather that causes strangers to smile at one another. Everyone looked carefree. They weren't worried about nursing or their newborn. They were enjoying themselves. People were sitting on the grass, riding their bikes, and making out on street corners. I was jealous.

By the time we arrived home in Brooklyn it was almost three o'clock. Anne helped us out of the car and was finally relieved of her duties. Six hours after Anne said she was going out for coffee, she waltzed back into her Wall Street office, coffee in hand, and sat down at her desk. No one noticed a thing.

Peter and I climbed our three-flight walk-up, a slow and painful endeavor. Regaining some of my strength, I insisted on carrying Sophie up the stairs. I held the baby as Peter unlocked our front door.

Now things would get better.

Chapter 3

The Panic and the Pain

I DIDN'T WALK through our front door and announce to our little baby, "We're home!" There was no time for tears or pronouncements. The rush was on to get organized before the next feeding. I had hoped I would cry, I needed that kind of emotional release, but it had been several hours since I last nursed Sophie. What I felt most when we arrived home was panic.

Sophie stayed asleep the entire car ride, the transfer to my arms, the three flights of stairs, and was still asleep when we lay her down in her crib for the first time. She was still a bit knocked out from her bout of jaundice. At the hospital Sophie had been fed every three hours. The pediatrician had given me instructions to feed the baby "on demand" or if she slept more than three hours I was to wake her for feeding. Sophie had been asleep for four hours. I knew that I should have woken her up, I should have offered her my breast, but I let her sleep. I wanted her to sleep for the next few weeks.

She was helpless and beautiful.

THE SUN streamed into our apartment. I pulled down the shades and closed the shutters. I didn't want anyone to see me nurse. I was full of milk and shame. And even though it was gorgeous outside, I never wanted to leave my house again.

The attitude of the nurses at the hospital didn't just make me feel like a novice. I felt like a dope. It wasn't that my know-it-all ego had been wounded. I was sucker punched by the learning curve. I had such a sense of entitlement when it came to nursing, which had gotten me nowhere. Why hadn't I solicited advice? Now I was home, and though I was still a new mom mess, I believed we had nowhere to go but up.

I decided to comfort my huge sore breasts before offering them to Sophie. The hospital's nursing handout suggested applying chilled cabbage leaves to soothe engorged breasts. Peter ran out and bought two heads of cabbage. He thought I was experiencing an odd craving, but he had learned long ago not to question the pregnant lady, which had now carried over to my new incarnation—the postpartum lady. We were lucky he happened to pick green cabbage. It is important to buy green cabbage, not red. As another new mom would later tell me, red cabbage stains everything. Peter pulled off two outer leaves, ran them under cold water, and brought them to me. I pulled down the panels of my nursing bra, removed the breast shells, pulled out a sample packet of nipple ointment, and smeared it all over my nipples. I returned the breast shells and then placed the leaves over my breasts. Cabbage supposedly has properties that work as an anti-inflammatory, and it did provide immediate relief. I'm not sure when Peter left the room. I think it was somewhere between the ointment and the cabbage.

While I was in our bedroom doing God knows what, Peter finally took a shower and changed his clothes. He straightened up the

44

apartment and unpacked our bags and the freebie diaper bag from the hospital. On the kitchen counter were the tiny cups to feed Sophie, formula, and those nipples.

Halley, who was still out in Long Island at my in-laws, wasn't our only pet. We also had two cats. It was because of them that we had purchased a glider and matching ottoman instead of a rocker. As our vet explained, rockers caused a great deal of cat tail injuries. The glider was comfortable and fit my romantic notions of motherhood. I also bought a heavy C-shaped Boppy brand nursing pillow, which Peter referred to as the "boobie." My nursing setup was a far cry from the uncomfortable and sterile environment of the hospital.

Sophie began to stir in her crib, and her noises soon turned into that newborn cry. There was no putting it off. It had been nearly five hours and it was time to nurse. I sat in the glider, wrapped the nursing pillow around my waist, and took off my many breast contraptions. The distance from my newborn to my breast was still uncomfortably far away. I hunched over. Sophie's crying got louder the closer she came to my breast. Her head moved side to side. I was sliding back and forth. The nursing pillow didn't have a flat surface. I spent a great deal of energy just keeping her from rolling off. Sophie's mouth tried to latch on, but there was nothing for her to latch onto. Flat nipples and engorged breasts created a latex balloon affect. Imagine trying to grab hold of a firm balloon with your mouth. I opted to pump a little and cupfeed her formula.

The thing was I was still a breast-pump chicken. I was unwilling to take the advice of the head nurse on the maternity ward. I didn't double pump. I was too scared to turn up the suction. Had I done both of those things, the pumping would have drained my engorged breasts, and draining is the name of the game with engorgement. I'm not advising you to turn the dial all the way up to the maximum, not at all. You could hurt yourself quite a bit with too much suction. But you need to double pump and you need to inch that dial up on the

Classic. I didn't even have the knob turned to the middle. It was practically at minimum pressure.

I kept thinking back to the one latch I had seen, in *The Blue Lagoon*. That baby just latched right on. That scene didn't look anything like the freakish performance I had going. That first day home I pumped and attempted a few more feedings that all looked and felt so unnatural I didn't see any hope in getting this nursing thing down. She was a tired little thing, but after she was fed she stayed awake for a little while. Peter and I took turns holding her. I loved her pouty lips, and the swelling around her eyes was beginning to fade. I dressed her in some of the fancier baby gifts and wished she didn't need to eat. When I wasn't trying to nurse her, I enjoyed our new mommy-and-baby moments, but I was relieved every time Sophie went to sleep and dreaded her next feeding.

Even though I had an appointment scheduled for the following day I had hoped to get another lactation consultant out to our apartment that night or early the next morning. My messages were panicked. "Hi, this is Lisa Shapiro. My breasts are getting huge and very hard. I need help. My baby can't latch on. I'm in pain. Please call me back. Would love to set up an appointment. Please . . ."

"Hello, I think I'm in trouble. My breasts feel like they may rupture. Please call me . . ."

It was late. Sophie was asleep and I knew it was time to put down the phone.

I woke up to a cool wet sensation on both sides of my chest. I had begun to leak milk profusely. Not only did I smell of cabbage, but now there was sour milk in the mix. It must have been three o'clock in the morning. I made my way to the bathroom and looked in the mirror. There I stood, puffy and swollen as before. I slowly peeled back the front panels of my bra. I took off the cabbage leaves and there they were, my gigantic breasts. They had grown several cup sizes. They were perhaps a D, far bigger than my usual B. In that light they looked like double D and felt granite hard. No longer round or breast-shaped, they now came to a point. Like Madonna's pointed Jean Paul Gaultier corset from the *Blonde Ambition* tour. But instead of cloth and wire, picture human skin.

"They are going to burst," I told myself.

I needed to have them surgically drained. There was nothing you could tell me otherwise. Maybe my breasts needed to be surgically removed altogether. My appointment with the lactation consultant wouldn't be for another thirteen hours. If I could get a doctor at the hospital to insert a needle and drain my breasts I would be relieved. The suction on the breast pump was foreign to me and I couldn't distinguish between discomfort and the new sensation. The idea of turning up the pressure was something I couldn't bring myself to do. The delivery was nothing compared to this pain.

I went into the kitchen and applied new cabbage leaves. There on the butcher block were the nipples the nurse had given us. Those nipples were begging to be used and there I was applying cabbage leaves to my *Ripley's Believe It Or Not* breasts. Not yet, I remember thinking. I wasn't going to reach for them yet. Though I was terrified by what I had just seen in the mirror, my determination was kicking in. Perhaps the hormones were fueling its strength.

Peter came into the kitchen. I must have woken him up. He looked at me and mimicked a drunken frat boy. "Hey someone's got big boobies."

"What did you say?" Peter opted for silence.

"Did you just say, 'Someone's got big boobies'?"

He nodded his head up and down. He looked frightened. He had done wrong, and he knew it. Peter was just trying to make a joke late at night. After all, his loving wife had been replaced by the engorged cabbage creature. Now the creature was pissed off.

"I just gave birth to your child, motherfucker. You got that?" Peter again nodded in agreement. "You will never . . ." I moved into within an inch of his face. "You will never ever make any comment about my breasts. Is that understood?"

Mute and scared, Peter nodded once more.

"You will never make a breast joke, a nursing joke, an engorgement joke. No more jokes. Not about boobies, breasts, melons, nothing."

He just stood there.

"You got that?" In tears, I went into the bedroom and pumped again. I worked up as much courage as I could and turned the suction up a notch. Squirts were coming out. This was an improvement. Sophie was still asleep and Peter was hiding somewhere in our two-bedroom apartment.

I REGRETTED missing that breast-feeding class. I kept thinking labor was the hard part. Everything after that was natural. It was supposed to be the most natural thing in the world. Breast ruptures must have been discussed in the class I never went to. On the chalkboard I bet the instructor wrote some statistic with the words, "In very rare cases" and next to it was "breast rupture." Like in the film *Scanners*, but instead of some guy's head it was going to be my breasts that were going to explode.

I was going to be a cautionary tale. And Peter would be sorry for that boobie joke.

Sophie woke up, not with a cry, but with a moan. The song in my head played my new nursing anthem. "When you walk through a storm keep your head up high . . ." I sat back in the glider and placed Sophie on the pillow, and once again I hunched over, she cried, and all I felt was pain.

I continued my routine of trying unsuccessfully to nurse Sophie. One lactation consultant returned my call and though she couldn't make it out that morning, she worked with me on the phone. She

48

told me right away that after hearing my message she knew I was going through "engorgement panic." She explained that engorgement panic is a condition where women are so distressed that they actually believe their own breasts are going to rupture. She assured me that no, that wasn't going to happen to me. I was advised to lay ice on them, which helped. I told her I already had a four o'clock appointment scheduled with another lactation consultant, and she told me the ice would help until then.

The rest of the day was a blur of monotony and discomfort. When Peter spoke to the consultant on the phone, she reiterated several times that we needed to have the baby hungry. If she was full or didn't want to nurse then the consultant wouldn't be able to help me. We decided not to feed Sophie after two-thirty that afternoon until the lactation consultant arrived. By four o'clock Sophie was awake. She was hungry, she was screaming, and the consultant was running late.

Around four-thirty we buzzed Laura in through the front door of our building. Ten minutes and three flights of stairs later she came into our living room. She could best be described as red. Her face was red. Her hair was red. She was breathing heavily and moved her head up and down to answer yes when we offered her a glass of water. She reminded me of an English professor I had in college, right down to her flowing linen smock dress. She must have been in her mid-forties but had a girlish face. Tucked under her arm was a large green pillow contraption encased in plastic. As Laura drank the cold glass of water my husband handed her, Peter whispered to me. "Don't buy anything." He wasn't sure if the whole consultant thing was a scam, and looking at that pillow I wasn't sure myself.

I prepared myself to go back to the hospital. I knew that I was a sorry case. Once Laura saw my breasts she would say, " My God, get an ambulance." Laura caught her breath and followed me down the long hallway to our bedroom. She was still bright red and for a moment I wondered if we would be taking her to the hospital.

I figured she had never seen anything as severe as my engorged breasts. I sat down on the bed and pulled down the panels of my bra. "Should we go to the hospital?"

She took one look and said, "You, I'm not worried about. On a scale of one to ten, you're a three."

"What does a ten look like?"

"You don't want to know. So, where have you been nursing?" I pointed to the glider. "Let's set you up on the bed." She began to build a platform for me on the bed. She placed two pillows against our headboard. I sat down and then she stacked two pillows on my right side and one pillow with two receiving blankets on top of that. Laura looked at Sophie in her crib. We had put a pacifier in Sophie's mouth so she wouldn't completely lose it before I had a chance to nurse her.

I could tell what Laura was thinking. "I just put the pacifier in because I didn't want her to scream, she's very hungry."

"A lot of times nursing moms get into trouble with pacifiers because it masks the signs of hunger. But it's not clear if they were already in trouble and used the pacifier or if it was the pacifier that caused the trouble. It's a good idea not to use them."

Point taken.

Next Laura saw a tube of breast ointment next to my bed.

"I've been using this because my nipples are sore," I explained.

"You know what works better? Soaking your breasts in warm salt water. Fill a coffee mug with warm water and add a teaspoon of salt. The problem with the ointments is that the pain you're feeling is your body's defense mechanism. It's telling you the latch is wrong. We see a lot of women get into trouble with the ointments. They'll keep smearing the cream on and in the end they haven't fixed the actual problem."

"But doesn't everyone have pain from nursing?" I believed the initial pain was unavoidable. Why else would they sell all that ointment if sore nipples weren't "normal"?

"Actually, if your latch is correct one shouldn't have pain." I was taken aback. I thought the pain one experienced from nursing was a rite of passage. As Laura dropped that bombshell, she took Sophie and laid her on my nursing pillow in front of me, adjusting the two receiving blankets under her head. It never occurred to me that nursing wasn't supposed to hurt. And who knew I wasn't supposed to hunch over? Why hadn't I thought to build a platform for Sophie? Laura now had Sophie completely in line with my nipple.

"You want her nipple to nose." Laura pointed to the direct line the platform created, which in fact did bring my nipple right next to Sophie's nose.

Laura also instructed me not to bring her into my breast directly, but to think counter-intuitively and aim her bottom lip to the bottom part of my aureole. The pressure from Sophie's bottom lip would turn my nipple directly into the baby's mouth. Laura used her thumb to show me. The baby was to latch onto the breast, not the nipple. Amazingly enough I saw how simple it was.

I explained how crazed Sophie became the closer she came to my breast. Laura explained that Sophie was what they referred to as a "frantic eater." Frantic eaters move their head from side to side, are anxious, and cry at the breast. It's just too much for them. Because Sophie was a frantic eater, Laura showed me how to wrap her up in a receiving blanket, pigs-in-blanket style. Laura folded the receiving blanket three times to create a long rectangle. Then with both of Sophie's arms securely by her side so she couldn't flail about, Laura showed me the proper way of getting her into a headlock. I wish I knew about this baby straightjacket sooner. Perhaps I wouldn't have bitten her in the hospital. I was lucky in one area of nursing: Sophie had no problem opening her mouth. She always opened up wide.

"She's cute," Laura said. For a brief moment I left crisis mode and looked at Sophie. She was cute. Her eyes were beginning to open and from time to time she peered out. She was so feminine. Perhaps it was because she wore pink from head to toe or the way her eyelashes seemed to curl upward.

"You must say that to all the new moms." I was trying to make some small talk. After all, this stranger I had known for only five minutes had just touched my breast.

"Actually, I don't. My father was a salesman. He went door to door, so he saw a lot of ugly babies. He told me the thing to say with an ugly baby."

"What's that?"

"You just say, 'Now *that's* a baby.' But she's really cute." Laura smiled at little Sophie. I made a mental note to watch out for that turn of phrase, and to use it in the future if need be.

"The hair makes her seem older." I was chatting up Laura. The more we talked the less I would have to nurse and by that Friday afternoon I hated nursing. "I had to wake her up last night after three and a half hours, but I think she would have slept longer. She seems like a sleeper. My mom says I was a sleeper when I was a baby."

All business, Laura turned back toward me. "That's great. Are you ready?" With Laura's hand guiding my arm she moved Sophie into my breast. It was a swift movement with the power to close a car door. "That mouth's open wide for a short time, so you have to move fast," Laura explained. Just before Sophie was completely hooked on, I pulled my body back.

"Wait wait, let's try again, I wasn't ready." I was afraid.

"Okay, ready?" Laura made the movement again pointing to Sophie's bottom lip and where on the breast we were aiming for. This time we made contact. We were using the transition or cross-cradle hold, which goes across the front of your body. And as the baby gets bigger, it's the most common position. It is sometimes described as belly to belly.

Though I was propped up with plenty of support, the actual nursing pillow made it difficult to keep Sophie level. I was using my arm to keep her from rolling off. Laura helped delatch Sophie, who was frustrated and crying.

"I hate this pillow," I told Laura. "She almost rolls off every time."

"This pillow works for some women, but with a newborn we recommend the pillow I brought."

"Can I try it?" I was willing to try anything.

"If I take it out of the plastic you're going to have to buy it."

"I'll buy it." I ignored Peter's earlier instruction. Out went the heavy nursing pillow. Laura slipped the new pillow out of its plastic casing. The tag read "My Brest Friend." Though I had seen the pillow in stores, the concept of having a "brest friend" kept me from buying it. Little did I know that in the months to come, the pillow would indeed become my best friend.

Laura attached the pillow's Velcro belt around me. With its large flat surface I no longer worried about Sophie rolling off and could concentrate on a good latch. Again Laura placed her hand against my wrist and together we brought Sophie in. This time she laid Sophie on the pillows she had placed next to me and showed me another position, known as the football hold, which is exactly what it looks like. I could score a touchdown with Sophie securely tucked under my arm.

It took tremendous concentration to keep my wrist straight. Sounds simple enough, but the natural reflex to bend my wrist was difficult to stop. I couldn't help it. I wanted her mouth to go over the nipple with her lips around the areola instead of using the pressure of her lower lip to bend the nipple into her mouth. It took several tries and every time I would bend my wrist at the last moment. The last try Laura kept a firm hand over my arm and together we kept my wrist from bending.

Sophie's lower lip was at the bottom of my aureole, just as Laura had showed me. My nipple bent directly in her mouth, her bottom lip was pushed on the outer rim of my aureole, to create a perfect latch. She was pushed in deep into my breast. Sophie drank away. She was gulping down and the swish and swallow were unmistakable. There was no question she was nursing. I could see the muscles in her neck move as she swallowed. For the first time since Sophie was born I actually heard her drinking from my breast. I was dumbfounded.

Poor little thing, five days of futile attempts and now she was finally drinking away. I was so thankful we cupfed her formula. She could have become dehydrated or malnourished otherwise.

I had never felt so inept.

Nothing the lactation consultant showed me was even remotely familiar. The whole process—not moving my wrist, bringing the baby in from the side, not aiming for the nipple, bringing her in deep into my breast—these were things I never would have come upon on my own. I was angry at those nurses at the hospital, not one of them had it right. I kept thinking about that first nurse squishing Sophie's face into my breast. What kind of instruction was that?

"Could I accidentally break her neck?" I asked.

"Everyone asks that question. No, you can't break her neck. See how her back is completely in line with your arm?" Laura pointed to Sophie's back and my arm, which were pressed together.

"Do you feel any pain?" Laura asked me.

"A little," I said.

"On a scale of zero to ten, zero being no pain, is it a five?" Laura needed a number.

"I think it's a three or four." I wasn't sure.

"Okay, let's delatch," Laura said. Laura told me to wet my finger, which made breaking the suction on the side of Sophie's mouth much easier. I had been delatching Sophie with a dry finger, which was uncomfortable and not that effective. Laura made me pay close attention to the way one's nipple looked when you delatch the baby. For the last few days my nipple had looked like a used-up lipstick with a point at the end, a sure sign of pinching. It is the pinching that hurts, and the result of the pinch, such as the pointed nipple, is an indication of an improper latch.

"Now let's do it again—we're trying for a three or under." Again we brought Sophie in and she drank away just as before.

Laura suggested pumping before each feeding in order to soften my nipple. That way Sophie would have an easier time latching on. To take the edge off Sophie's hysteria I would cupfeed her several ounces of pumped breast milk or formula before each feeding as well. Then I would wrap her up in a receiving blanket so I could get a good grip. And at about ten miles an hour I would bring her into my breast in one swoosh. The promise of easy nursing wasn't going to be fulfilled anytime soon, especially with a fifteen-minute warm-up just to nurse. But I'd gladly take pain-free over easy at this point. If I stopped nursing then I would still be in pain and engorged for days, which I calculated would be about the same amount of time to achieve painless nursing.

"Are my breasts going to get softer?" I asked.

"In about twenty-four to forty-eight hours your breasts are going to feel softer. They're not going to feel like your old breasts, but they'll be softer. The key is to get a good latch so the baby can drain each breast fully." She went on to explain that I should alternate breasts at the start of each feeding, start with the left in the morning, next feeding start with the right. Newborns will usually need both breasts at each feeding, but they will nurse more from the breast they start with. Lastly, I was instructed to pump after each feeding if I still felt full. Laura prepared a work sheet that listed positions, which pain levels were too much, and when I should relatch.

I regretted waiting so long for a session with a lactation consultant. Much of the pain I had experienced was unnecessary. I definitely needed another session. Laura got on the phone and arranged an appointment for Sunday morning. I had to go the next forty-eight hours alone. She didn't work Sundays, but assured me that I would be in good hands with her associate Ilana. Somehow I knew Laura wasn't going to climb our stairs again.

Before Laura arrived, I had secretly hoped she would discover something that would make nursing impossible. She would tell me I had an infection or the baby would never learn to swallow, though both of those conditions are not reasons to stop nursing. But at the time I didn't know that. Instead I was told Sophie was an efficient and good eater and if anything I was overproducing milk, one of the better problems to have.

When Laura left I felt better.

"You bought the pillow?" my husband said without disguising his true feelings that somehow his wife was a sucker in some huge nursing scam. Remember this is a man who did not know breast pumps existed until that week. Not the most knowledgeable person when it came to breast-feeding. I think he was surprised by all the stuff I needed to breast-feed. The new pillow pushed him over the edge.

"Yes, I bought the pillow. It's so much better." I gave him my best don't-question-it look.

Peter took another approach. He was supportive and thought better than to give me a hard time about the pillow. He kissed me. "I'm so proud of you for trying to do this." I was touched, but part of me still thought he was buying some time before my next freak-out.

I was amazed at how I actually had to be shown how to nurse. Unlike that idyllic photo from the breast-feeding pamphlet, my look was a little different. I had my baby in a receiving blanket straightjacket and headlock. My hair, which was not washed, was up in a ponytail. Cabbage leaves poked out of my big nursing bra, which concealed my plastic nipple protectors and nursing pads. Instead of the rocker, I sat on the bed with some kind of man-made pillow attached to my waist. The pillow was reminiscent of the old cigarette boxes women wore in speakeasies while shouting, "Cigars, cigarettes." That was my motherly image, and I'm not even going to talk about the granny panties.

Chapter 4

They Are Going to
Reach Out and Touch You

BEFORE I HAD SOPHIE, the mirror had been a place to pluck eyebrows, check for blackheads, and blow-dry my hair. I mixed lipsticks with a brush and penciled in the outline with a corresponding color. I curled my lashes and in the full-length mirror I tried on outfits, while asking the cliché, "Does this make me look fat?" Now I couldn't bear to see my face, all puffy and red. The appearance of my breasts, large and pointy, was revolting. But there was another image.

After Laura left, I caught my reflection while walking past the mirror in our living room. I was holding Sophie. I had to stop and take it in for several minutes. Though my face and body were swollen, that image of me holding a baby, my baby, in my arms was novel and romantic all at once.

I was a mommy. With all that had happened in the last five days, that idea of me being a mom was all-powerful. It trumped the giant breasts and chipmunk face. Holding Sophie while standing in front of the mirror was a refuge from nursing.

The other truth about nursing was it called for good hand-eye coordination.

Athletic ability never came easily to me. I smashed my thumb the one time I caught a fly ball in Little League. In my four years throwing shot put I placed only once by way of forfeit. I wish I had been better at shot put. I couldn't help but think athletic women around the globe were nursing with ease. I became competitive with myself, saying over and over in my head, "I am going to get good at this." I focused on Sophie's lower lip, trying to bring it toward the edge of my aureole. I would get it wrong and off she'd come. It was a rare latch that succeeded on the first try.

Later that night after nursing Sophie it happened.

A tiny drop of blood appeared on my left nipple. That was the moment I feared. I had read about cracked nipples in the hospital's handout. With that tiny blood blister, I was sure cracked nipples would be my next mishap. It had been only a few hours since the lactation consultant had left. I had the new pillow. But now I'd hit blood.

I called the consultants' twenty-four-hour help line. Laura was on call, and she instructed me to pump on the left side, giving the breast a rest from nursing. Next she told me to soak my nipple in warm salt water. I filled a coffee mug with warm water and about a teaspoon of salt. I bent forward, placing my breast into the mug and stood up straight. The salt water didn't leak. I had created some kind of breast/coffee mug vacuum. It immediately brought relief. Later I moved up to two to three teaspoons of salt, but this isn't advised. I soaked each breast for about five minutes, then placed the plastic breast shells back over my nipples, the breast pads over the shells, and finally applied two well-chilled leaves of cabbage on top of that. All I needed was special sauce and a sesame seed bun.

I fed Sophie on my right using the football hold and then cupfed her a few ounces of formula and pumped my left breast. If you are going to cupfeed it is important to pump so your output is close to or equal to the baby's intake. Each feeding took about five minutes of prep time, fifteen minutes on the actual nursing, and fifteen minutes of cupfeeding and pumping for a grand total of thirty-five minutes. I would have anywhere from an hour to a three-hour break. Then the whole process would start again. That is how newborns nurse. There is no breakfast, lunch, and dinner for them. It's just feeding upon feeding; it's normal but overwhelming.

NOW THAT the weekend had arrived, we began having visitors. This took some planning. I had to wear a shirt big enough to conceal the cabbage and all my nursing contraptions. I would socialize for about half an hour. If I went longer than the thirty minutes my body allowed, I ran the risk of leaking through my breast pads. So I was careful to excuse myself, change, and return long enough to say my good-byes.

I know I wasn't the prettiest picture of new motherhood. I could see the surprise in people's faces when I opened our front door. "Wow, *look* at *you*," a family friend exclaimed upon seeing me. And I can only speculate on how I sounded. With each visitor I opened up about my nursing problems. I had the urge to tell all. I played a role in my nursing drama. I should have read more, asked more questions, and been better prepared. The price for those mistakes had been high, which left me fearful of my own body. When rehashing the last few days' events, I was torn between confession and caution.

Several people handed me the most lovely baby gifts. There I was opening up a box containing a hand-knit sweater or booties and I would just start talking. "Oh this is gorgeous. Did you make this? I am so touched. Can I tell you, I am having such trouble nursing. I love the color. Did you ever nurse? Because I had no idea I had flat nipples. Oh, look at these buttons, they're little puppies, how cute. You see I got engorged. I thought my breasts were going to rupture. Oh, is this the matching hat? I love that *(short pause)* and I have a blood blister on my left nipple. Did you know you could put cabbage leaves on your breasts to reduce the swelling? I can't image being one of those women who love to nurse. You know, who really has issues? Those women who nurse until their kids are four years old. I am just going to nurse for a little while, and it's solely for the health benefits, that's the only reason I'm nursing."

I'd look over at said visitor's face and they seemed disoriented and would say something like, "Did you see the card?"

"Where are my manners? This card is so cute," I would say, opening the card last. "You know those women who nurse forever, why? Why would anyone want to do that?" I tried hard to concentrate and read the card, but it was a jumble of letters to me. My comprehension had been shot days ago. "Thank you. Breast-feeding is gross, sticky, and smelly. You know it caused me terrifying pain. Did I tell you I bled?"

"Yes, you mentioned that." For whatever reason, none of our visitors were able to stay too long.

WHILE THE health benefits were a big part of my motivation, what really propelled me in my quest to nurse was ego. Most of my friends and family knew I was nursing. It was all so public now. In the wake of my massive missteps during Sophie's first week of life, I had become driven to succeed.

What I couldn't rectify or understand was how could nursing be easier? If Sophie was on formula I could be out getting my nails done. I could have a baby sitter watch Sophie during the day, which would have given me a much-needed rest.

The leaking drove me crazy. There is a muscular ring behind the

60

nipple that can be loose or taut and that is why one leaks or doesn't leak. It was luck of the draw about those tiny nipple muscles. Eventually they become fully functional and one's leaking is lessened or ceases altogether; until that time I wore pads. I drenched about ten pads per breast per day. Often I'd leak through my pads and would change my hideous bras several times a day. I just dripped, leaked, and even sprayed. I didn't understand exactly what was going on. And I still didn't own a real book on the subject of nursing. I had spent the two weeks before I had Sophie making lemon bars for my husband and lip balm for friends with my new Martha Stewart Lip Balm kit. Perhaps I should have spent my time more productively reading up on mammary glands and the like.

I later met many women who owned several books on breast-feeding long before their babies were due. And by the end of that first week of Sophie's life I should have sent Peter out to buy a book. I had been too overwhelmed. I could have ordered one from Amazon or from one of the many breast-feeding Web sites, but there were too many options. I didn't even have the presence of mind to ask Laura to recommend a book. I think I also resented the pamphlet and handouts I had received. I resented every pregnancy magazine I ever read.

I thought of those ubiquitous warning signs, the ones about pregnancy and alcohol consumption. There should be a big warning label like that in every new-mother magazine and pamphlet, but instead of the alcohol warning it should simply read, "If you are going to nurse, seek the help of a certified lactation consultant within a day or two of giving birth." If there was anything I really needed to read it would have been that.

WE WERE trying to cut down on the amount of formula we were feeding Sophie. Now that I was successfully pumping I was trying to give

Sophie only breast milk when I cupfed her. Each day I cut down on the supplemental formula while adding to her intake of breast milk.

I tried to focus on what I was feeling at each feeding. On a scale from one to ten, what kind of pain did I feel while I nursed Sophie? My nipple was still coming out white and a little pinched after each feeding, and whenever I nursed her on one breast, the other breast would leak ounces into my nursing pad. I'd end up heavily soaked after each feeding. My breasts were still lumpy and hard, but I was thankful that they no longer felt like stone.

ON SUNDAY MORNING Ilana came through our front door. Ilana had a fair complexion and light eyes. She smiled like we were old friends. Immediately I wished she were an aunt or close relative. After the cursory introductions we got right to work. I was sitting on the couch in our living room and had several pillows adjusted around me to give the right support. Now that I understood the fundamental nipple to nose concept, the platform to prop Sophie up was easy to assemble. I had "My Brest Friend" attached around my waist and had placed a pillow behind my back to keep it straight. Two pillows were put to my side for an armrest, and several receiving blankets were folded into squares to bring Sophie's head level to my breast. I also had my feet up on a footstool. As Laura had explained, your knees should be above your hips. That way you are able to sit up straight. Comfort and avoiding a nursing backache were easy now.

"I can't get the latch right, and now I've hit blood," I explained. "I also think Sophie has diarrhea."

"What does it look like?" she asked. "Is it mustard colored with what looks like seeds, sesame seeds?"

"Exactly," I told her.

"That's what a breast-fed baby's bowel movements are supposed to look like. If it was diarrhea it would go right through into the diaper, there wouldn't be anything on the surface."

"I had no idea." And I didn't. It had looked like diarrhea.

"May I?" Ilana asked before moving in. One thing you have to get over when you work with a lactation consultant is that she is going to touch you. She is going to reach over and hold your breast in different ways. Ilana looked very closely at both breasts, paying careful attention to my left nipple.

"I had a tiny needle-size blood blister there." I could no longer see where the blood blister was. "Now I'm just pumping on that side."

"It looks like it's healing."

Her first suggestion was to wrap Sophie not in a receiving blanket but in a large-size square cloth diaper, not the rectangular padded kind. She folded the diaper several times. It was less bulky and therefore I could handle Sophie better. Ilana also suggested aiming my nipple for the roof of Sophie's mouth. It had the same result as aiming Sophie's bottom lip for the edge of my areola, but for some reason that concept worked better for me.

"I'm nearly four ounces ahead of her now," I said. Ilana reminded me that over-producing was a good problem to have.

"Why is over-producing considered a good problem?" I didn't understand the idea of a good problem.

"Because it is easy or relatively easy to fix. When women don't produce enough milk, which is less common, you need to work with tubes, pump often, and supplement. It can be much more involved. For you, soon you'll get in sync with Sophie's needs milk wise." I was assured that over time Sophie would be less frantic, I wouldn't be as engorged, and at some point in the near future I wouldn't be bothering with cupfeeding or pumping. I would latch her on every time she was hungry and she would nurse. That was the goal.

Ilana did an evaluation of Sophie's sucking. She covered her index finger with a tiny latex cover and put it into Sophie's mouth. Immediately Sophie began to suck. Sophie did have a slightly tight frenulum, which is that stringlike tissue that connects the bottom of your tongue to the bottom of your mouth. To this day, frenula are sometimes cut because they are too short and can get in the way of nursing, but Ilana didn't think that was Sophie's problem. The problem wasn't her sucking and it wasn't my milk supply. It was the latch.

"Okay, you want to bring her in so I can see how it's going?" I began to bring Sophie in and Ilana watched closely.

"Try and hold your breast like this." She made the letter "C" with her thumb and index finger and demonstrated a better way for me to hold my breast. The thumb went above the areola and the index finder went below, giving it extra support.

We covered the same territory as with my visit with Laura, but I needed another run-through. Because Ilana appeared to be without judgment, I didn't hide my frustrations each time I had to relatch. I was exhausted. I had lost my bravado after that first night in the hospital. What Ilana saw before her was an angry mess.

Fifteen minutes into our first session Ilana asked, "Do you want to pump, and just supplement with formula?" That was my out. She had seen my struggles and hesitation. It was validation. I was allowed to quit.

Perhaps if I had been asked a day or two before I might have opted out, but not now. I had seen too much progress. I had seen and heard my baby drink and swallow. Sophie was on with a low pain level of about a two.

"Let's try again."

"She's eating beautifully," Ilana offered. There was a certain rhythm to her eating. She would start out fast and furious and would wind down to a steady slower pace. Sophie nursed away for several minutes. My breast felt like a deflating water balloon, which Ilana assured me was a very good thing. She confirmed Laura's observation; Sophie was efficient and I wouldn't have to spend as much time nursing.

After Sophie nursed a while, but clearly wanted more, we delatched her so we could practice bringing her in again. When Sophie wasn't anxious for another gulp I tried to buy a little downtime by asking a variety of questions about nursing.

"I've heard that what you eat affects the baby. Are you supposed to stay away from chocolate?"

"Studies have indicated that the mother would need to eat something like a pound of chocolate to make an impact on the baby."

I mentally reviewed my apartment, where the chocaholic's equivalent of a keg party had taken place. The empty two-pound box from Bon Bons was still on the kitchen counter. Out on our dining room table was the remainder of what was a milk chocolate assortment from See's picked clean of everything but the nut chews.

I didn't pursue the subject any further. Sophie was beginning to fuss and some things are better left unanswered.

I latched Sophie on several more times. Sometimes I felt a pinch while other times I didn't. Even when I didn't feel a pinch, my nipple would come out with a pointed tip. It was obviously pinched, which made me wonder if I had any nerve endings left.

"Okay, you're still getting a pinch. It may be her way of controlling the flow. If the milk is rushing out, she may be using her tongue to slow it down. That may be why you're getting the pinch." Ilana held Sophie and looked into her mouth again.

After our session I asked Ilana, "How could women think this is easier?" I took my six-day-old daughter out of her headlock and unfurled her.

Ilana took a neutral position. "Well, for some women it is. They don't have to clean and carry bottles with them, and there are benefits to nursing. Studies prove that children that are breast-fed are less likely to get sick, so you don't have to take care of a sick child as much. You save money on formula."

"What is the minimum amount of time you need to nurse for a baby to get some kind of benefit?" I asked Ilana.

"The recommendation is six months for certain health benefits, but there are studies that show a baby has a reduced risk of ear infections after four months." Ilana filled out a new work sheet for me. I later read online that The American Academy of Pediatrics recommends breast-feeding for a year and The World Health Organization's recommendation is even longer.

I figured I would try to make it through the next four months and then wean Sophie.

We made a plan. When my left breast looked better I would try to nurse Sophie on it once a day, adding another feeding each day after that.

"You may want to come by the breast-feeding support group that's held on Wednesdays. It's just a couple blocks away at the hospital." Ilana handed me the work sheet, which reiterated her suggestions for the upcoming feedings.

"Is it one of those groups where everyone talks about how much they love breast-feeding? I don't want to be around *those* women. I heard about those women who love to breast-feed and nurse for years," I went on. "I just don't think I can relate."

"A lot of the women are there because they had similar trouble learning to nurse their babies." Ilana was the group leader. Besides, she explained, "It's free." Considering a lactation visit was costing over a hundred dollars, the idea of a freebie was appealing. I told Ilana I would come to the group, and in the meantime we scheduled an appointment for the next day.

"Look," I said, "she's a very strong baby." Sophie was holding her neck up on her own, if only for a few seconds, not bad for a six-day-old.

Ilana said, "She gets that from her mother." She smiled as she left our apartment. Sitting there on the couch with my nursing pillow still in place I realized how desperately I needed a compliment. I would have paid a hundred bucks for that comment alone.

THE TRUTH began to come out from others in the next few days. Any friend or relative who told me they nursed got a litany of questions from me.

"How long did you nurse? Did you supplement with formula? Did you nurse through some sheet of plastic known as a breast shield? Did it hurt? Did you ever pump? Were you ever engorged?"

The answers revealed the big truth, or more appropriately, the big lie. My husband and I once visited a couple who claimed nursing was going great, yet their little one was drinking twenty ounces of formula a day from a bottle. Not exactly an accurate account of nursing. I received an e-mail from a friend who admitted that it took three months for her to get nursing down, and for a while she pumped pink milk. All that and she never sought the help of a lactation consultant. It turned out that the several relatives who claimed to have nursed only did it for a week. Others supplemented heavily with formula or nursed through plastic shields. There was even a woman I knew who lent a battery-powered pump to a girlfriend. After the girlfriend's nipples cracked, the friend admitted the same thing had happened to her using that *same* pump.

More than sex, more than money, women I knew and respected lied when it came to nursing. I still don't know exactly why this was. When a woman claims that she nursed her baby, that's usually the end of the conversation. People in general are not familiar with nursing. It's not out there in our culture. Science has proven it's the very best thing for a baby. Why not lie? There isn't anyone around

67

to call her bluff. I promised myself that I would never lie about my nursing experience.

ASIDE FROM the new revelations made by friends, relatives, and acquaintances on the subject of nursing, there were lots of first-time introductions as we showed off Sophie. I was lucky so many people brought food. I was always hungry. Someone even sent me a make-your-own-cannoli kit from the Termini Brothers of Philadelphia, one of the better gifts a new mother can receive. Another couple brought us trays of food from Artie's, the Upper West Side deli. I gorged myself on macaroni salad and pastrami sandwiches. My sisters brought pints of Ben and Jerry's Peanut Turtle special edition ice cream. My parents and in-laws brought dozens of gifts and more macaroni and cheese. Since word spread of my cravings for my comfort food, there had been a macaroni and cheese bake off of sorts.

Lucky for me, I was a nursing mom and little Sophie needed me to eat away. In the end, it would all be nursed out, I thought.

In those first two weeks home I left the apartment only once. We went into the city for Sophie's one-week checkup at the pediatrician. That was it. Sophie had gained a half pound, which was good news considering all the trouble I had had nursing her. I weighed myself as well. I had dropped fourteen pounds since Sophie was born. My all-you-can-eat diet seemed to be working.

When we returned home, it was time to feed Sophie. Peter went out to run some errands. Now I was alone. I sat down at my designated spot in the living room, feet up on stool, My Brest Friend snuggled around my waist, and Sophie in her carefully wrapped position. I latched her on correctly the very first try, which was a rare occurrence. She nursed away, gulping furiously at first and settling

68

into her slower rhythm after that. Sophie came off all by herself. My nipple came out perfect. Completely content, she fell fast asleep. I pulled her into my chest, wrapped both arms around her, and burst into tears.

Chapter 5

Get Yourself to a Breast-feeding Support Group

THE NEXT WEDNESDAY, I put on some makeup, did my hair, picked out my big blue Egyptian cotton work shirt, and prepared to head out to the breast-feeding support group or "breast support group" as my husband called it. Sophie was two weeks and two days old. I weighed myself again: My total weight loss since Sophie was born was twenty-six pounds. Considering I had gained forty-four pounds while pregnant, I figured I was halfway there. Since it took me two weeks to lose all that weight, I figured in just two more weeks I would be back to my pre-pregnancy weight. I gave myself the once-over in the full-length mirror. Even though I had lost weight I still looked fat. I feared running into someone I knew. I was certain they would think I had let myself go. If only I owned a shirt that read, "I'm not fat, I just had a baby." As long as I pushed the stroller and kept the baby close to me, my appearance would be understandable. I decided that I would not, under any circumstances, leave the house without the baby. Everything would make sense with a baby in my arms. She wasn't an accessory but an explanation.

Peter was looking over our new stroller one last time to make sure it was set to go. It was one of those big multi-functioned strollers, the SUV of strollers. Yes, we lived in a three-flight walk-up. No, I never bothered to stop a mom in my very mommy neighborhood in Brooklyn to ask, "What's the best stroller for this environment?" Common sense could have come into play with a simple word problem. If you live on the fourth floor, should you buy a forty-pound stroller that is difficult to collapse, or an easy eleven-pound stroller?

Remember, it is always the childless who become first-time mothers. The segment of the population least equipped for the job gets the position without even an interview. Yes, you may have had that baby-sitting job all through college, but anthropologically speaking we were supposed to have witnessed a thousand latches by the time we had our own offspring.

I was thankful Peter had taken two weeks off from work. Everything was a production, from changing a diaper to maneuvering the stroller out of our house. If ever I needed my husband, it was during those first two weeks.

Out we went. I was still wearing the plastic breast shells. They made me even more self-conscious, like Barbarella, only chubby and unsightly. My poor nipples were still recovering from that first week of bad latches. Though Sophie was allowed to nurse from my breasts, no one, not even myself, was allowed to touch my nipples, not even by accident. They were officially quarantined from all non-baby contact.

It was my first real outing. I looked forward to seeing Ilana. I could show her my latch and she could tell me how my nipples looked. Ilana had come to our house three times in the last week, so we were already on an every-other-day schedule.

Now I was in the process of extending the days in between visits and slowly weaning myself into independence.

Peter walked with us all the way to the hospital's fourth-floor maternity ward, where the meeting was being held. We said good-bye.

I was out in the world again, this time with a baby. After ringing the bell several times, I was buzzed through to the maternity ward's prisonlike security door. A small windowless classroom next to the nursery was the designated meeting place of the breastfeeding support group. I had visions of strident "Nursing Nazis" sitting around at the meeting. "Nursing Nazis" are those mythic creatures you hear about on the news or through friends, the ones who are arrested for nursing their ten-year-olds at the mall. I once saw a woman who could best be described as a zealot. She was being interviewed on a prime-time news magazine. The interviewer asked her what she thought when she saw a baby drinking out of a bottle. She said, "I think yuck. When I see a baby drinking from a bottle I just think yuck." Her voice was nasal. Her tone was harsh. The next shot had her nursing her son on a park bench. He looked old, four or five, possibly more. She looked down at him and said, "Are you getting enough?" When I saw that clip, and it was years ago, I remember thinking yuck.

Though I never actually met a "Nursing Nazi," I was loath to meet anyone who would utter the phrase, "I love nursing my baby."

I was fifteen minutes late, but the meeting was casual enough that no one seemed to notice. The classroom had half a dozen nursing pillows, a large hospital-grade pump, and posters along the wall with slogans that read "Fast Food Outlets, Two Convenient Locations," "For a Healthy Baby, See Attached," "Kids Eat Free," and "Suck Up to the Boss."

There were several moms with babies who looked six or seven months old. That's right, they had been nursing for that long. It was unfathomable to me. The other women weren't puffy and swollen. They wore casual clothes, their hair was done, and their bodies looked fit. They looked together. I wished just for the purpose of blending in that there was another new mom with a newborn. Ilana told me that there usually were several newborns at the meetings. I was anxious to commiserate with my own kind. She assured me that most likely there would be a new mom at the next meeting.

Ilana set me up with one of the hospital's "Brest Friend" pillows. I sat in a chair and we wrapped Sophie up in her diaper. She looked like a tiny mummy. I held her in my own type of death grip and brought her in. If her head moved so much as a millimeter off, I would get a pinch. Sometimes on the news they show military footage of jet fighters refueling in mid-air. That's what latching Sophie on was like. It took precision. It took complete concentration.

And then came the sweat. You will never sweat as much as you will when you first start to nurse. It is a sweat beyond Nixon, beyond the flop sweat that Albert Brooks experienced in that scene in *Broadcast News*, it is a sweat beyond any send-up of an antiperspirant commercial. You'll be changing your shirt as often as you change diapers. My advice, which I should have taken that day, is to wear clothing that doesn't change color when it gets wet. A baggy white T-shirt will hide the outpouring when in public. My crisp blue Egyptian cotton work shirt turned into a modern abstract painting soaked with cobalt blues. Forget the armpits. My body liked to create two wet pools, one under each breast. The hormones that let-down your milk also trigger the sweat, and stress exacerbates the problem.

Then there's the thirst, which goes beyond your wildest dreams. Pre-baby it is difficult to imagine how thirsty you will become. Always have water nearby when nursing. A good bendy straw isn't a bad idea either. I was so thirsty that I actually contemplated buying one of those novelty hats that support two cans of beer. The ones that read something like, "I've got beer on my mind." I'd throw two bottles of spring water where the beer should go. But Peter had already seen me with a nursing pillow strapped around my waist, not to mention the cabbage and the breast shells, and I worried that the novelty beer hat would have sent him packing.

At the group, with my sweat and thirst in high gear, Ilana and I went over Sophie's latch. Ilana thought there was definite continued improvement. She also felt the time had come to remove the breast shells. In many ways, the direct pressure they placed on my breasts was contributing to the profuse leaking.

"I'm amazed you're out of your house at two weeks. That's great," Stephanie, a mother of a six-month baby boy, told me. Mother and son had matching dark brown eyes and light brown hair. "At two weeks I couldn't leave the house. I had so much trouble nursing and I didn't get help at first."

Another woman who looked to be in her late thirties was sitting crossed-legged on the floor with her large baby girl across her lap. She wore her long blond hair up in a ponytail and was dressed in a loose-fitting T-shirt. On her right hand was a carpal tunnel splint. I, too, was wearing my cuffs because the pain in my wrists had yet to go away. It wasn't a good sign to see the mother of a seven-month-old still wearing hers. But what was most surprising was the necklace-type contraption called a supplemental nursing system, which she wore around her neck. The small square plastic container was filled with formula or breast milk. A tiny clear tube went down from the container all the way to her breast and was taped to her nipple. Apparently she never produced enough milk and was still supplementing. I avoided looking at her directly, but it was difficult not to stare. I thought back to my conversation with Ilana about being an over-producer and how that was an easier problem to fix.

The woman noticed my carpal cuff and told me that even though her daughter was seven months old, she still needed to wear the cuff when she nursed. We both realized we shared the same natural childbirth instructor. I confessed that I went drugs all the way.

Her name was also Lisa and her story was more harrowing. Two weeks past her due date, her dreams of natural childbirth were dashed when she was induced and eventually had a C-section. Her

74

story gave me some perspective on my own hell at that moment. If this woman could nurse her baby using a supplemental system for the last seven months on top of a C-section, it was time to count my blessings as an overproducer. She had taken the breast-feeding class. I asked her if she thought the class was any help.

"I got some good advice." She shifted her daughter and the clear tube to her other breast. "I was told that it takes six to eight weeks to get nursing down. But then it gets easier." There it was, that word again, "easier." At first glance nothing about her nursing her daughter looked easy, but unlike me, she didn't seem stressed or pained.

I was now so soaked with sweat I felt compelled to bring it up. "I can't believe how much I'm sweating. And I'm so thirsty."

"It's the hormones, it won't always be like that. I remember being drenched the first month," Stephanie said.

"Would you care for the pillow?" Ilana asked the woman sitting on the floor.

"OK, I'll break down and use a pillow." The woman using the nursing system gave in. That was the other thing that amazed me. How could anyone nurse without the pillow? It was almost a status symbol. Those who can go pillowless were the pros. I resolved to be rid of "My Brest Friend" soon. I would be pillowless in a matter of weeks.

The other plus to attending the group, aside from meeting other nursing moms, was the fancy digital baby scale. I weighed Sophie. She had gained nearly half a pound since last week. Sophie looked healthy, no longer yellow from jaundice. As the meeting was emptying out, I placed Sophie back in her stroller.

"We meet every other Wednesday," Ilana reminded me.

I turned the conversation back to my favorite topic, myself. "Great, you know I just lost twenty-six pounds. It's coming right off," I bragged.

"That's wonderful, because a lot of women hit a plateau." I didn't really register what Ilana was trying to tell me. Peter arrived.

He stood back from the meeting room's door and just waved from the hallway.

"Everyone left, I'm the only one still here. You can come in."

"I'll wait out here." Peter would never again be in such close proximity of the breast-feeding support group.

As we were leaving, a maternity ward nurse stopped us.

"Could I see your paperwork?" She sounded official.

"No, she's two weeks old, we were just here for the breast-feeding support group." I pointed back to the meeting room.

"You know you both looked a little too together for new parents, a little too well-rested, but I wasn't sure." The nurse laughed. I was thrilled someone would actually mistake us for being *together*.

"Has she had one of those giant BMs yet, the type that gets on everything? They're explosive." This was small talk on the maternity ward.

"Not yet." We left the hospital.

Two blocks and the power of suggestion later, we used an entire box of baby wipes to clean up the biggest, most explosive bowel movement any baby has ever made. There would be many more.

Before we made it home, we stopped by the pharmacy to buy every stain remover available. I waited out front while Peter went inside. Standing outside the pharmacy with our giant stroller on the corner of Pacific and Court, several moms zoomed by with their light urban Macleran strollers. They were moving at a fast clip. I wasn't sure if it was from a passing car, across the street, or one of the moms who blurred by, but someone yelled out, "It gets easier!"

It must, I thought.

Chapter 6

Feed unto Others as You Yourself Would Like to Have Been Fed

BY MID-MAY it already felt like summer, though it was difficult for me to distinguish. Our apartment retained an intolerable amount of heat. I experienced what felt like a hot flash every time I nursed. Peter bought two new air conditioners, now we had one for every room. If you have a spring or summer baby and can afford it, get air-conditioning, or central air if possible. On that first hot day I took on a new look. As Peter pointed out, "I never thought you were one of those walk-around-in-your-bra types." If I had taken up smoking and playing solitaire I would have made the full transformation into one of Marge's sisters on *The Simpsons*. I didn't look celebrity new-mom good and nowhere near the terrific image I fantasized about.

Sophie was three weeks old and aside from her red-and-pink skin tone, she didn't look like a newborn anymore. Gone were her swollen pugilist's eyes, a souvenir from my hour and a half of pushing. Looking at photos taken just a dozen days before, I was amazed at Sophie's makeover from newborn to infant. It all happened so fast. Make sure you take lots of photos and video, they change almost by the hour.

We were fortunate that all of our immediate family lived within an hour and a half drive. With Peter back at work, my mother helped out several days a week. My younger sister's summer job fell through and she, too, was available to babysit. Between the warmer weather and a bout of apartment fever I made a conscious effort to get out more. My mother and I strolled all around my neighborhood. The fact that our destination of choice was to the newly opened Ben and Jerry's was beside the point. With nursing using up all my calories, I was sure the five-block walk would do away with any brownie sundae residue.

We lived in an older part of Brooklyn. The big slate squares that made up our sidewalks were uneven. I had to watch my step even without a stroller. The wayward roots of trees had snagged my heel on more than one occasion. Sophie was jostled to sleep every time we went for a walk, which wasn't a bad thing. It's just that her tiny head was still floppy and every once in a while I would think it flopped a little too much.

My mom and I became backseat stroller pushers. "That's too bumpy," I'd say.

"Watch her head," she would tell me. Peter and I played the same roles on our walks. At first I went slow, stopping often to adjust her hat or check her blanket. I was doing what my father-in-law referred to as *mishing* with the baby. It's a Yiddish word that means to mix or in our case to fuss. "Stop mishing," Peter would say, having adopted the line as his own.

Finally on one of our outings, the owner of our local deli walked by. "You're never going to get anywhere if you keep stopping like that." He was right. From then on I tried to keep a steady pace and stopped only if it was completely necessary, which was often.

78

BEFORE I had Sophie and even during that first week, I had spoken with my mother only on a superficial level when it came to nursing. Her comments had been supportive. They were all along the lines of "You'll be fine." "It's the most natural thing in the world." I didn't believe she was being dismissive. My mother-in-law told me she had forgotten all about nursing and I assumed the same was true for my mother. One of my few friends with children confessed that she had blacked out the first six months of both her sons' lives.

I had never heard my mother speak about nursing as being difficult or painful. I was impressed that she nursed me without incident and much of my determination to succeed at nursing was fueled by the nursed baby's Golden Rule—feed unto others as you yourself had been fed.

The fact that I was a breast-fed baby was something I had always taken for granted, but now I appreciated what my mother had done for me in a whole new way. We had had a tenuous relationship over the years. But with the arrival of Sophie my mother and I found common ground and enjoyed each other's company.

There hadn't been a great deal of time to reflect those first few weeks. But on my walks my mind had the luxury to drift. I kept thinking about what Ilana and Laura had gone over with me, that my engorgement didn't have to be as severe as it was. Had I latched Sophie on correctly from the start I wouldn't have gone through the panic and the pain.

"I didn't have to be as engorged as I was," I told my mom.

"Mine were like rocks. They were huge." My mother held her hands in front of her chest like she was cupping imaginary DDs.

"It must have hurt." I knew from my own experience that if they were big and hard, my mother must have been uncomfortable. It was difficult for me to relate to my mother as a new mom. She had been so young, only twenty-one years old when she had my older sister,

Anne. At the time she was living in South Africa, a hemisphere away from family. "So what did you do? How did you get help?"

"I nursed you all, and I tried with Anne. But she was impossible, I couldn't get her to nurse." She stopped. "I was so embarrassed. My breasts were so big. They offered me a pill and I took it. It was this pill that dried up my milk. So I gave Anne formula. My friend told me, she said, 'Lucy, you can get your milk back.' But I was just too embarrassed."

My mother stopped walking. Her gaze seemed more focused. She had remembered, remembered something from those days.

"You told me you nursed all of us." I couldn't hide my surprise.

"I did, but I only nursed Anne for a few days. And I would have nursed Edith longer but she had a severe allergy to my milk, to the point where we found mucus in her stool. The doctor convinced us to switch to formula. But I think I should have tried to change my diet first. I ate a lot of hot fudge."

"Wait, wait, was I nursed?" Confused by these revelations, I needed to know if I had been nursed. At the time I thought my mother was combing her memory but she was really looking for the right choice of words. "Mom, was I nursed?" I asked again.

"Yes of course you were nursed. You were nursed for six months. I wish I had gone longer." She paused. "You were the only one I really nursed successfully. I was able to latch you on right away and I was staying with Mother. I guess I had more confidence and I was *determined*. You weren't even twenty-four hours old when I brought you home. You nursed right away and I never got engorged."

"How come you told me you nursed Anne? Why didn't you tell me you got painfully engorged with Anne?" Now this is where I could have said, "Oh really, you got painfully engorged, hmmm . . . information I needed three weeks ago!"

However incredulous I felt at that moment, it turned into something else. I felt sad for my mother, for how young she was, and how embarrassed she felt. It was heartbreaking. Instead I readjusted Sophie's blanket.

"I didn't want to discourage you," she said, staring at Sophie in the stroller.

I've had this internal debate ever since my mother told me her logic about not warning me about engorgement, about her own initial failure with nursing, and about keeping her nursing story from me. There was a time, soon after our conversation, that I had felt betrayed, that she should have told me all of that before I went into labor. I believed she owed me that. I theorized that I could have lined up an appointment with a lactation consultant the day after delivery, that I would have read more, and been better prepared. But as the shock of her full disclosure subsided and time passed, I have come to the conclusion that in many ways she did the right thing. Had I known that she had given up with my older sister, I believe I may have seen it as my own escape hatch of sorts. "Well, I could always succeed on the next one," I would have told myself as I reached for the formula.

Later I would ask Laura her position regarding the ethics of what to tell or not tell children about being breast-fed. It was Laura's professional opinion that mothers should lie. "If one child was breast-fed and the other wasn't, we advise mothers to tell them that both were breast-fed. Otherwise it tends to create jealousy and resentment." Laura's answer made sense to me.

Yes, I wish I had known genetically speaking that I could be predisposed to overproducing milk and I should have been on the lookout for certain problems from the get go. If you can, it helps to find out your mother's nursing story if she has one *before* you give birth. But this is not always possible.

And though my mother couldn't give me instruction or practical advice about nursing, she had been nothing but supportive. During Sophie's second week she even gave me a gift certificate for a lactation consultant visit. What a great new mom gift. And I was lucky. I had heard and would hear many more just-give-him-the-bottle stories about those mothers or mothers-in-law who discouraged their daughters from breast-feeding. What new mother needs that?

"I just didn't want you to give up," my mother said, and with that we walked into Ben and Jerry's.

I WISHED my mom had had the access to a group like the breast-feeding support group. There I had a point of reference. I wasn't the worst breast-feeding mother in the world and my problems weren't unique. I didn't intend to miss a single meeting and had marked every other Wednesday on my calendar for the next two months.

My nursing and pumping styles were evolving. At Ilana's urging I recently attempted double pumping, and it did make a huge difference in the amount of milk I was able to pump. I had a greater letdown and expressed more milk—ounces more. Since we were still cupfeeding Sophie, I tried to give her only expressed breast milk instead of the formula. With double pumping I almost had enough.

IN A DIRECT reaction to my mom's story, I felt possessed to warn my friends about the pitfalls of nursing. I knew several pregnant women and decided to call each one to give them a giant heads-up about nursing. It wasn't that I had regained my know-it-all footing, there was something else at play when it came to women and nursing. I couldn't put my finger on it. By explaining my troubles, my friends could all learn from my tale and it would prevent them from making the same mistakes.

My first call was to a friend in LA. Her baby boy was due in three weeks.

"Hey Jennifer, it's Lisa, not sure if you're still working, but call me. I have to tell you all about nursing." I was sure I would hear from her right away after leaving that life-altering message on her voice mail.

Two days later she called me back.

"Hey how are you doing?"

"Good, just three more days left here at the office."

"Listen, do you plan to nurse?"

"I'm going to nurse exclusively for a year." Jennifer was so on the ball, her emphatic answer spoken in the nursing vernacular made me feel foolish for calling.

"I had some trouble, I got tremendously engorged. I had difficulty latching Sophie on, it was really hard and you need to get the help of a lactation consultant because you're not going to know if you're in trouble until the twentieth feeding, and you absolutely have to rent the Medela Classic, and if you can, find a group that meets, like a breast-feeding support group."

"Yeah, I'll get that to you right away. Lisa, sorry someone just came into my office. Yeah, I have a pump, my friend lent it to me. From what people tell me, everyone is different." I felt like a complete jerk. Obviously not everyone was in the dark with nursing. I wondered if I would have heeded the same warnings if someone had called me with all that unsolicited advice. And Jennifer seemed prepared. She already had a pump, and I was amazed by her commitment to nurse, "exclusively for a year." I questioned my commitment to nurse for just four months. How could anyone nurse for a year?

I was sure I would hear from Jennifer when she got into trouble. How could a woman not have trouble? "Well, if you do have any trouble, feel free to give me a call, I went through so much." Stepping outside of myself, I must have sounded like a freak to Jennifer. Calling her at work with my Chicken Little the-sky-is-falling scenario.

Jennifer never did call. We received a birth announcement but no calls. Much later when I called her she told me she had given up on nursing after a few days. She never saw a lactation consultant, and her only real comment on the subject was defensive. "Not everyone has an easy time like you." It was obvious she hadn't heard or more appropriately hadn't listened to anything I had told her. I changed the subject.

Chapter 7

Behind Every Successful Nursing Mother

ILANA made her last visit to our home that third week. I looked forward to every visit as a way for me to judge the ever-evolving progress.

"Looks like you're doing very well."

"You think?" I still needed "My B*rest* Friend" pillow, I still used both hands to nurse, one to bring Sophie in and the other to support my breast.

"See I can't latch her on and nurse her like the photos in the magazines." I gestured to the way my thumb and index finger still needed to support my breast or Sophie would pop off. "You know how you see women just cradling their babies in their arms without having to support their breasts?"

"Sometimes women can do that because they have an older baby or because their breasts are smaller. Sophie still needs the support because you're breasts are long."

Long.

Long wasn't exactly the adjective I would use to describe my breasts. They were full, round, pretty, and in their former life were a 36B. Not a 36B Long.

In my third week progress was slow. I was still pumping, cupfeeding, and pinning Sophie's arms to her side with a cloth diaper. Every feeding took a good deal of preparation. Sophie also had a habit of falling asleep in the middle of a feeding. I would place her back in the crib and an hour later she would be back on the breast. Ilana thought Sophie was what is referred to as a "cluster feeder," meaning that she would nurse a great deal for several hours, literally tanking up on milk. A cluster feeder will nurse on demand, with the feedings becoming more frequent in the evening. From six in the evening to around ten she seemed to feed nonstop. Even if I fed her twenty minutes ago, the second she'd fuss I'd offer her the breast and she'd nurse some more. There was a huge payoff to all that nursing. She slept. She slept all night.

"Now you need to just keep feeding her the way you are." Sophie was nursing quickly and without interruptions. I could hear the gush of milk hitting the back of her throat. Then she would take a giant gulp. "Look, she's eating beautifully. What a pleasure." Nursing wasn't exactly a pleasure for me, but anything that was pain free began to feel like bliss. I did take pride in every ounce Sophie gained and just holding her was a pleasure. And I was also convinced Sophie had smiled at me.

I had hit a new nursing plateau of sorts. Until Sophie grew a little bigger and my breasts were a little softer, there wasn't that much more Ilana could do. I wasn't in pain. I didn't have a breast infection.

"Should I make another appointment?"

"Why?"

"Just so you could check up on me."

"Come to the meeting next Wednesday, call me if you have any trouble before then, but at the meeting we could go over whatever you want."

"Also, do you think insurance covers lactation consulting? Should I submit the forms to my insurance?"

"Some companies cover it and some don't. We recommend that you send it in and see what happens." It was hard to believe that lactation consultants weren't automatically covered. I submitted my paperwork and figured at least some of the visits would be covered.

"You know I wanted to ask you one thing, I almost forgot. My left wrist is killing me. They put the IV in right where it hurts, but I'm not sure if it's because I had carpal tunnel syndrome when I was pregnant. You know I still need to wear the cuffs."

"You should try wearing the cuffs when you nurse. They can help keep you from bending your wrist when you bring her in. Try that. See if it helps." I kept thinking about the woman I had seen wearing a carpal splint while she nursed her seven-month-old at the group. Was that going to be me?

"You know I always latch her on better when you're here."

Most new moms I knew agreed with this observation. Feedings always went better when a lactation consultant was in the room. It was true at the support group and it was true in my own home, the feedings always went smoothly. This last visit I noticed that I was doing all the talking. It was a running commentary. "See she isn't pinching as much." Or "Now watch as I delatch her." Ilana was patient and watched. Our session was short and before I knew it Ilana packed up her bag. She checked her pager, returned a call, and headed for the front door. I would see her at the next breast-feeding support meeting, but what lay ahead of me was practice.

As uncomfortable as I was at the idea of anyone seeing me nurse, my resistance to cooking was even greater. When Peter came home I announced that it was a perfect night to dine al fresco. That meant packing up the "My B*rest* Friend" pillow, which I planned to use if Sophie needed to nurse. Sophie was three weeks old and thus far I had been able to avoid any public nursing. I had packed the pillow every time my mother and I took a stroll but luckily Sophie hadn't wanted to nurse, was asleep, or we put the pacifier in so I could make it home. Yes, we had used the pacifier. There were times when we needed it.

We loaded Sophie into the super tank. Later, when I grew tight with my mothers' group, we all confessed to owning some inappropriate piece of baby equipment. Turns out I wasn't the only one with the giant stroller. Along the way to an Italian restaurant we passed several women with older babies and toddlers. Once again they all seemed to speed up as they walked by.

An inside table might have provided more privacy, but we chose a table outside for the breeze. My sweat glands were still in overdrive. With our stroller and diaper bag, we took up a lot of room for two people and a baby. It was just past six o'clock so we were the first ones there. The key to dining out with a baby: Get to the restaurant early. The earlier you are, the more accommodating they'll be.

All through dinner Sophie slept soundly. The rickety walk to the restaurant had lulled her to sleep. I ordered salad, pasta, and garlic bread. As usual, I was famished. With all the water I was drinking I also had to go to the bathroom constantly. It wasn't as often as when I was pregnant, but it was more than my pre-baby self. I excused myself to the ladies' room.

There really isn't a right time to bring this up, so now is as good a time as any. I was so focused on nursing and my breasts that all else seemed secondary. But I was still tender from my tear. And so I used a spray bottle filled with water to take care of business in the bathroom. I brought along Tucks wipes, which are soaked in witch hazel, to use if things got more involved. I cannot speak in terms of recovering from a C-section, but if you had a vaginal delivery you may want to pack a little kit that you can take along to the bathroom. That's what I did. I was also wearing maxi pads. At first I wore them with the disposable underwear I stole from the hospital. And as things lightened up, I was able to wear the granny panties, and slowly made my way back to thongs, but that takes time. You're not going to be wearing a thong for a while.

Midway through our dinner I noticed I had difficulty pulling my bread apart. Earlier that afternoon my left wrist had gone from annoying ache to throbbing pain. I took a Motrin. In the hospital I had been allowed to take Motrin even though I was nursing. The Motrin also helped with the new achey sensation I felt in my breast. It was a tingling feeling and if I was distracted I could ignore it, but if I paid attention the sensation made me crazy. Had Ilana not seen me earlier that day, I would have been worried that I had a breast infection. She explained that the pins and needles sensation was the feeling of my milk coming in. As Sophie's needs grew, my milk supply grew as well.

There I was at our favorite outside-patio Italian café eating my angel hair pasta. All seemed well with the world if I could ignore my breasts and my throbbing wrist. At least Sophie remained asleep. I wasn't ready to nurse outside with "My Brest Friend" pillow, not that night. Sophie began to stir.

"Check please." I would nurse her in public, just not yet.

THE NEXT MORNING I told Peter, "I'm going to call my doctor. I think I sprained my wrist."

"Let me know if you need me to come home." Peter left for work. Though I had the help of my relatives at least twice a week if not more, I was on my own with Sophie that day. I called my doctor. The fear that something was wrong with my wrist was terrifying. I had

89

come so far nursing Sophie. I didn't need another obstacle to overcome. The list already included flat nipples, engorgement panic, frantic eater; was I going to add a sprained wrist to the mix? Convinced my problem was connected to the IV they put in my arm, I swore I would never have an IV again.

My doctor could see me if I could make it to the office within the next two hours. She was located near my Midtown office, which was great when I was working, but now on maternity leave the schlep into Midtown seemed impossible. Peter would have to come home, watch Sophie, and cupfeed her breast milk if she was hungry. If he ran out of breast milk he would have to give her formula. It was still too early to give Sophie a bottle. Since Sophie and I had had so much trouble getting our latch down, I didn't want to take a chance with nipple confusion.

I hoped to return home within four hours' time, which was about my limit. After that I would have to nurse or pump or risk becoming painfully engorged. The plan was Peter would then go back to work. In retrospect it would have made sense to take Sophie with me, but I still needed so much stuff to nurse her—the pillow, the cloth diaper wrap. The whole breast-feeding process was more freak show than womanly art. I feared getting arrested for child abuse if someone witnessed me latching on my daughter.

I tried to dress in something slimming, which entailed wearing a long skirt with a big sweatshirt tied around my waist. Who did I think I was fooling? I wore my dark sunglasses and hoped I wouldn't run into anyone I knew. It was odd to get on the subway. My last months of pregnancy had been a world of car services. It was strange pushing my way through the turnstile. "I haven't been here in ages," I thought. I was in a living flashback to my pre-baby self. I hadn't properly prepared for the trip either. I hadn't brought water, and I was already thirsty, and I didn't bring anything to read. It was my first moment in a while to do nothing.

90

The train came right away. I was going to make good time. That first time I was out and about without Sophie was an out-of-body experience. It felt familiar but everything had changed. I had nursed Sophie less than an hour ago, but my breasts were already filling up. Self-conscious about their size, I felt all eyes were focused on them. Could anyone tell I just had a baby? I wondered what Sophie was doing and if she was crying or still sleeping.

The doctor's waiting room had tons of magazines. I could finally catch up on current events. There I was reading an old *Newsweek* with newfound passion. Just what the hell was going on in the world? They had *Business Week* and *People*. That was the life, sitting there reading magazines. I was just waiting and doing a little bit of nothing. Doing a little bit of nothing was for the leisure class, which was how I now referred to those without children.

The medical technician called me into the examining room. While waiting for the doctor, I slid off my flip-flops, and got on the scale. I hadn't dropped a single pound in the last week. How could I still weigh 174 pounds? I was twenty pounds away from my fatty weight. "How can that be?" It made no sense. So much milk was flowing out, how could I weigh the same? It crossed my mind that perhaps I wasn't going to lose all my weight without trying, but I dismissed it. Next week I'll weigh myself and see where I am, then I'll worry.

The doctor's appointment went pretty much how I imagined. She had no idea what was wrong with my wrist and gave me a referral to see a specialist on another floor in the building. She could try and get an appointment with him that afternoon. I knew my breasts were becoming engorged, but I also knew that my wrist hurt, especially now since I was focused on it. It was a roll of the dice, would I be able to see the doctor before the pain in my chest outweighed the pain in my wrist?

I took the elevator down to the hand specialist's office. I got past the officious secretary and sat down on the waiting room's plush sectional sofa. Several plaques lined the walls, all etched with his name

91

and various awards. His waiting room was packed. I had hardly noticed the pediatrician's office located down the hall, but now all I heard were the cries of babies. The wail made my milk let-down. I was wearing pads in my bra; going without breast pads wasn't an option for me. If you do have the propensity to leak, make sure you travel with extra pads, a half dozen just in case of an emergency. I had stashed four pads into a Ziplock bag before I left. Nothing could be worse than leaking in public. I went into the bathroom and changed my pads. The way I was leaking, it occurred to me that four might not be enough. I took my seat in the waiting room and again, my milk let-down. There must have been quite a few babies at that pediatrician's office, and they all seemed to be crying. Sitting around reading magazines isn't as fun when you're subjected to that strange-baby-crying milk-letting-down torture. After about an hour, my name was called.

The hand surgeon was well groomed. I on the other hand felt one breast pad away from a breast milk let-down breakdown. I told him my story. He examined my hand, which didn't appear swollen. I had X-rays taken and waited for the results. All the while I looked at my watch. It had been nearly four hours since I last nursed Sophie. My chest was rock hard and sore. I hadn't been this engorged since my first week. I kept thinking I would be home in an hour. I called Peter and told him the same thing.

"The tendon is definitely swollen," the doctor told me.

"What do you think it is? I had an IV go in there, and now I'm nursing all the time. I had carpal tunnel in both wrists while I was pregnant and I still have it."

He looked closely at the X-rays. "I can give you a shot of cortisone now, and I can give you a splint to support the wrist. Until you stop nursing there isn't that much I can do."

"If you think the shot will help. Can I nurse with the splint? It won't be too big?" I had tried to nurse Sophie with my wrist supports but found them bulky.

92

"After you leave here, just walk down the street and they'll fit a splint for you. You have a pretty common nursing injury."

A nursing injury?

That's right, the doctor told me I had injured myself nursing. I had a nursing injury.

I was so bad at nursing I had actually injured my arm. True, he mentioned something about hormones in the body, retaining fluid, that my body still considered itself pregnant, or something like that. It was difficult to pay attention with the never-ending echo that played over and over in that hollow chamber that once housed my brain: "You have a pretty common nursing injury, nursing injury, nursing injury . . ."

I was worried that I wouldn't have the time to go down the street and get fitted with a splint. I had to make a choice between the pain in my breasts and the pain in my wrist. The wrist won. I was there and since I'd already cost Peter half his workday, I might as well get the splint for my "nursing injury." I couldn't believe it. I left with my prescription for a wrist splint. I walked into what looked like a hand-and-arm splint factory, took a seat, and waited my turn. I was glad to be free of the sound of crying babies. How cruel was that? I figured if I could get a cab right when I left the splint place, I could theoretically be home within an hour. I told the woman who fitted my splint to my arm how important it was that I would be able to nurse while wearing it. She didn't see that as a problem. When she fit the nine-inch plastic splint on my wrist and lower arm I thought there would be no way I could nurse tender little Sophie. How could I? They gave me cotton gloves to wear under the splint.

"You can wash these in a washing machine because they're going to get dirty." She leaned in close and added softly, "They tend to smell after a while."

With my new splint and "wrist socks" in tow I went out onto the sidewalk to hail a cab. In New York City there is the taxi witching hour when cabs look like they are "in service" but really what their light means is "off duty." All the cabs seem to switch shifts at the same time, which in the evening was right about the same time I left the splint factory. It was ugly. I gave it a solid thirty minutes and made a panicked call to Peter. I could hear Sophie's cry in the background.

"Where are you?" He was having his own private hell as well.

"I can't catch a cab." Just like that I was sobbing. I was helpless and my breasts hurt. "I'm going to take the subway." I pulled myself together, walked several blocks, got on the express, and found myself home forty-five minutes later.

I stormed into our apartment and took her at once. I strapped on the pillow, wrapped her up, and brought my little egg roll into me. She drank away to my great relief.

"What are you wearing?" I guess Peter hadn't seen it all yet.

"I have a common nursing injury." My splint bumped Sophie's head. She immediately cried and came off, but I latched her back on.

"How am I going to nurse with this?" I was tearing up, like when you don't want to cry and you have trouble seeing through those little pools collecting in your eyes before they exit in the long stream down your face.

Peter did what he had been doing for the last three weeks when I needed a hug, but was too encumbered by all my nursing para-phernalia to be physically hugged—he walked over with a cold glass of water, bent the bendy straw, and held it to my lips.

I WAS STILL too sore in the chest area to put Sophie in a Baby-Bijörn. I wasn't even willing to experiment with the baby carrier. It was bad enough that I had to wear a bra twenty-four hours a day just to keep my breast pads in place. Sleeping on my side was out of the question. I could maintain some level of comfort laying flat on my back, but if I turned, ouch. Sophie had slept nearly a six-hour stretch that third week. God must have taken pity on me. Look at her breasts, okay, let her little one sleep through the night.

Since I wasn't ready for the carrier, every time I left the house was a production. My mother came to help the day after I had been diagnosed with my nursing injury. I was in need of sympathy. And so we did what we usually did, we took an afternoon stroll.

On our way home from Ben and Jerry's we saw a brand-spanking-new mom along with several people who looked like her family, and the new baby. I was so excited to meet someone who was a first-time mom like myself. I introduced Sophie, my mom, and myself. Her name was Dena. She was a heavily made-up petite woman with spiky blond hair and retro eyewear. She told us her delivery had gone well.

"Are you going to be nursing?"

"Yes, exclusively for a year." There was that statement again, exclusively for a year. Where did they all get that?

"I have an amazing lactation consultant."

"I already saw one at the hospital." Dena was so together. She already saw a lactation consultant. At the hospital no less. Why hadn't I done that? Her little boy was sound asleep, but it was obvious his lips were severely dry and chapped.

"His lips look a little chapped, I guess you want to go nurse." Who the hell was I? Here she was bringing her new baby home and some stranger tells her that her baby's lips are dry and chapped so she should go nurse. "I mean I had so much trouble in the beginning, I got really engorged." I was trying to make up for the chapped lips comment.

"What's that?"

"I wasn't latching her on properly and my breasts filled up with milk, they got huge. I had engorgement panic and actually thought they could burst."

"Ewww . . . I didn't have that." Dena might as well have said, "Ewww . . . I didn't have lice." Or "I didn't get the cooties like you."

I assumed I deserved that for the dry lip comment so I held off telling her that it was day three for her, too early to tell if she was engorged. She wouldn't know if she was engorged until later that night at the earliest. Why had I been so open about my engorgement? Now I felt not so much like a cautionary tale, but more like a freak. Dena was about to go back inside with her newborn when her husband came out. His name was Frank and we congratulated him on the new baby. He was a slight man, who was impeccably groomed, right down to his overly trimmed mustache and tailored Oxford shirt. He seemed dazed, like a new dad.

"I'm starved. I'm going to go get a sandwich." Frank headed down the street toward the deli, not looking back at his wife or new baby.

"Could you get me one too?" Dena called after him. It wasn't clear if he heard her.

"You know next week there is a breast-feeding support group that meets at the hospital. Call me if you're interested or if you run into trouble or just want to hang out." Who wouldn't want to go to the breast-feeding support group? I wrote down my name and number.

Dena's baby started to fuss. "Gotta go."

We said our congratulations one more time and headed back to my apartment. I wasn't sure if I would hear from her any time soon. I knew I came on a little strong. It was difficult for me to hide my desperation. I wanted camaraderie. My mom focused on another aspect of our encounter. "Why couldn't he have offered to get *her* a sandwich?"

I DIDN'T hear from Dena.

Maybe she looked at the splint on my wrist, the funny looking pillow stashed in the basket of my stroller, the boxes of nursing pads one could see through the not-quite-opaque CVS shopping bag, and those large inescapable breasts pointed awkwardly out from my chest. Who would listen to me? I was grotesque.

The following Tuesday I left my mother-in-law Nola with the baby and headed out to have my highlights done. Not only had I chosen a difficult-to-style layered cut, but my blond highlights required a touch-up every two months at the least. If you learn nothing else from this book, I beseech you to have an easy hairstyle. Easy does not mean short, it just means that you should have your hair in a way that if you don't make it to the hairdresser's for the first few months, you'll still look okay.

I had pumped before I left and figured that at worst, I would fill up uncomfortably. I was going to a local place so I could always dash home if that happened. I ran into Dena and her husband, Frank, out with their new baby boy. Though he weighed in around six pounds those two weren't at all hesitant about stuffing the little thing into their baby carrier. Aside from being wary of putting Sophie in the carrier because my breasts were sore, I also was hesitant because of the product's minimum weight restriction, which was eight pounds. Didn't they read the warning label? And why was I being so judgmental? Was I actually that hurt that the only other new mother within a five-block radius hadn't called? Was I being hard on them because her husband didn't offer to get her a sandwich? And again, who the hell was I?

"How's it going?" I tried to keep a tight lip on any of my nursing gospel.

"He's latching on great!" Frank boasted. He was wearing what looked like an ascot, though it could have been a neck scarf. It was difficult to tell because of his jacket.

"Wow, that's amazing. I had so many problems." Had I not been to the breast-feeding support group, that comment would have really killed me. When did nursing get competitive?

"He just latched right on." I could tell there was a certain smugness at play.

"You guys are amazing, out here with your son. Well, if you're at all interested, I'm still going to the breast-feeding support group tomorrow." Frank began to walk on.

"Really? What time?" Dena didn't seem as cheerful as her husband, though she looked amazing for a new mom. She even wore eye shadow.

"It's at twelve-thirty. If you want I'll pick you up on the way. But you're lucky, you're not in any pain."

"Well, I have a little soreness," she said quietly.

"Come on," Dena's husband called over to her.

"What do you mean? I thought he was latching on great?"

"It's a little pinched." I had no idea why Dena hadn't called.

"Well, does it look like a worn lipstick?" I had learned to talk in those terms with the lactation consultants.

"Yeah, it comes out pointed." Dena seemed anxious.

"Well, that's a pinch, that means the latch isn't right. Look, do what you want, but if you can, I would go to the group. It's free and a lactation consultant runs it. Didn't you have a lactation consultant in the hospital?"

"Yeah, she said he latched on great."

"Sophie and I still need to do all sorts of things to nurse. We still cup feed her breast milk and formula before each feeding just to take the edge off. And Peter cupfeeds her at night while I pump. She took in five ounces last night."

"I mean I'm not *engorged* like you." She remembered that about me.

"Dena, we gotta go." Her husband rushed her along.

"Who knows, you may see me there," Dena called back as she took off down the street to catch up to her husband. He seemed to be scolding her, though they were too far away for me to hear. I turned around and continued walking.

I heard many bad husband stories during that first year. They were apocryphal tales told through the rumor culture of new motherhood. I heard the one about the new dad who spent his entire paternity leave playing *Grand Theft Auto*. There was the one about the husband who wouldn't let his wife see a lactation consultant because he didn't want to shell out the hundred and sixty-five bucks for an appointment. And the classic tale of spouse sabotage, the guy who says, "Just give him the bottle."

Behind every successful nursing mom is a supportive partner or friend. I may have been engorged, I may have leaked, I may have had a nursing injury, but I had an encouraging husband who believed in what I was doing. As I walked on to my hairdresser I had one thought on my mind. I was so glad I married Peter.

Chapter 8

Find Your Own Kind

I KNEW being the first in my circle of friends to have a baby was going to change the dynamic of my friendships. I just wasn't prepared for how much. Most of my girlfriends, the ones I went drinking with back in my pre-pregnancy days when I had the nickname "One-Chardonnay-Shapiro," were still single. When my single friends came to visit my newborn and me, I thought they were coming bearing gifts and to see how I was. But they really came to say good-bye. I know what you're thinking, "not my friends." Things change after you have a baby. Take my advice, start chumming up to the people you know who have children, they can help. All your single girlfriends will be able to do is make you feel fat.

Living in Brooklyn with a baby didn't necessarily put me in a leper colony, but it might as well have. I begged people to come out to see me. Often friends would ask, "When are you coming into the city?" For many it was their first trip to an outer borough. Before the baby, birthdays, bars, and get-togethers were all appropriately planned in New York City proper, Manhattan. Now I was giving long, involved directions that sometimes included a subway change.

Three girlfriends planned to visit at the same time. They had already canceled once. I had been so desperate for visitors that I'd cried with disappointment. I was starved for some good old girlfriend time, like the conversations I used to have right before I left work, or over drinks in the evening. Finally, when the weather conditions were right, they came en masse to Brooklyn. I noticed that my friends liked to travel in groups. That way if they got lost on the F train they could take turns short roping each other back to Manhattan.

I was the friend who just had a baby who was having trouble nursing. I was a novelty in their lives. Who knows how I sounded, on the phone, in my e-mails? I went on and on about the crazy contraptions I needed for my breasts and to nurse. Looking back, I know it was scary stuff.

Their visit had been timed so they wouldn't witness me nursing. Once they arrived I made room for them on the sofa. I literally moved "My B*rest* Friend" pillow to make room for my former best friends. I believe one of them asked, "What's that thing?"

"It is my nursing pillow," I answered. I would have been open to share more, but that was the last question any of them asked. Sure there would be phone calls and e-mails here and there with lines like "How's it going?" but they were all a year or two away from marriage, planning their next bicycling tour through Europe, managing several suitors, and reserving their place for a share in the Hamptons. I must have looked like their worst soccer-mom nightmare.

Many companies make hip comfortable maternity clothes, but I found it difficult to find anything flattering or remotely fashionable for that "transition" period after the baby is born. Big and baggy was what I wore. Before, I had rationalized that my big tummy was all baby, somehow without the baby it became baby fat. The more people who visited the more self-conscious I became. Not a single soul said, "You look terrific." And you know why no one said that: because I didn't look terrific.

After an hour, which must be the legal limit for single friends to visit with their married friends with babies, they would make up an excuse about a place or appointment they had. I was glad I had film in my camera to capture those last moments.

As they left, I heard them in the hallway through our walk-up's soft echo, "So where do you want to go now?"

I wanted to yell, "Hey wait for me." But it was too soon to leave the apartment for an evening out. My lactation consultant recommended waiting five or six weeks before trying the bottle so nursing could be well established. I couldn't leave Peter to cupfeed Sophie through an evening of cluster feeding. Also I hadn't been invited.

After my girlfriends left, I went to nurse Sophie and wondered what my friends were doing in the parallel universe of the childless. Were they all drinking? Were they meeting up with their respective boyfriends? Or were they all chain smoking away, discussing their own desire never to "breed"?

I felt as though I no longer had my place. Not with my old friends or with the other mothers I saw in the neighborhood. There was no new-mom welcome wagon, unless you count the barrage of junk mail I received from formula companies "welcoming" me to their club. Much later I would come to understand why moms with young children do not introduce themselves to brand-new moms. But at the time I just thought they were ill-mannered and mean. They must have seen me.

In some kind of trickle-down effect my cats were demoted as well. Our dog was spared this neglect because he was staying with my in-laws. But since Sophie came home from the hospital our cats had been starved of emotional attention and received only reprimands when they tried to sleep in the activity rocker. Sophie was now a month old and I couldn't remember the last time I had pet my cats. In an act of empathy, and perhaps a little solidarity, I played with them using the wire cat dancer toy and fed them a can of real tuna. "I know just how you feel," I told them.

I was eager to find my own kind.

IT WAS drizzling that Wednesday so I put the plastic cover over the stroller. And then, for the first time, I left the house on my own with baby Sophie. I was finally going solo. The trip no longer seemed momentous.

I navigated the slow-moving electronic super-sized revolving door, two elevators, and many corridors of the local hospital. I pressed the button to be buzzed in with a certain no-this-isn't-my-first-time know-how.

Once in the room I could see there were at least a dozen moms, three times as many as at the last meeting. And as Ilana had promised, there were several new moms there as well. There was even a line forming to use the digital scale. Ilana asked me about my wrist. Several moms wanted to know why I was wearing a splint. "Nursing injury," I told them, going on to explain the sore tendon and the carpal tunnel I had while pregnant.

I asked Ilana with a newfound confidence for a "Brest Friend" pillow. The hospital kept several in the breast-feeding room, but unlike my cloth-covered version they had washable plastic covers so they could be kept cleaned. Remember, nursing mothers tend to sweat. I recognized Stephanie from the last meeting. "How's it going?" she asked.

"Better." I took the seat closest to Ilana.

The chairs were arranged in a large circle, college seminar style. Several women taped tubes to their nipples that led to their supplemental nursing systems. There was one mother of two, a toddler and a newborn. She was preparing to nurse her newborn while her

103

toddler played around at her feet. Ilana was occupied placing the mother's tubing in the correct position so she could nurse. I learned that women use tubes for many reasons. Some women use the supplemental nursing system because of a low milk supply and one mother I knew used the tubes for a brief period in the beginning to strengthen her baby's weak suck. By her son's fourth week she was off the tubes and nursing exclusively.

"I think you could try a wider tube, see you're using the thinnest one." Ilana took a tube from a plastic bag and the woman attached the wider one.

I was busy wrapping Sophie up in her cloth diaper. I wasn't superstitious about nursing. It's just that the obsessive-compulsive aspects of my personality were rearing their ugly head when it came to "preparing" to latch Sophie on. My back needed to be straight. The pillow's Velcro needed to be strapped tight, my knees pressed together, one folded receiving blanket was under head. In my mind I was performing my own routine: "Brest Friend pillow fasten?"

"Check."

"Arms tucked tight on both sides of baby."

"Check."

"Folded receiving blanket under her head."

"Check." It was as close to working a pit stop or launching a rocket as I would get.

"Why don't we go around the room?" Ilana motioned with her hand to a young woman sitting to my left. She had long black curly hair and wore a vintage print skirt with a long-sleeve top. The woman looked fabulous. Her daughter had dark black hair and light brown eyes. I was taken out of my little world when I heard the woman tell everyone the name of her baby.

"I'm Rachel and this is Sophie."

The woman sitting next to her laughed.

"This is Sophia. You're the first Sophie I've met."

"You too." Rachel seemed surprised.

Everyone got a good chuckle when it was my turn. "I'm Lisa and this is Sophie."

"Is it Sophie on her birth certificate or Sophia?" Rachel asked.

"It's Sophia." I had an odd feeling in the pit of my stomach. Being a Lisa born in 1969 gave me intimate knowledge of what it was like to live with a common name.

Was this just coincidence? Was it a one-time occurrence with the name I loved and chose for my daughter or did I inadvertently name my daughter the Lisa of 2001?

"So we have three Sophies here." Ilana laughed. As I brought Sophie in she made her usual grunts and moans. The Murphy's Law of nursing, the quieter the setting the louder the sounds Sophie made.

"She used to make all those sounds when she nursed." Rachel pointed to her Sophie. "Do you have any nicknames for her?"

"Sophieofi, that's what we've been calling her lately." I could only think of one. Peter and I hadn't explored nicknames for her yet, it was too early in the game. Though she would need a nickname soon if I ran into any more Sophies.

"We call her Sofa, Sophiesofa."

"She has lots of hair, too," I said, pointing to Rachel's daughter.

"My pediatrician said Sophie was the only baby she ever saw with a perfect part." It was true, her baby's hair parted a little off to the side. "It looked this way the day she was born."

Several women were late. I didn't see Dena enter the room, but noticed her when she took her seat behind Ilana.

"Glad you made it," I mouthed to her. I had regretted telling her about all things nursing, so I felt somewhat relieved to see her there.

"How old?" another mom asked Dena.

"Ten days," Dena replied. The younger the baby the more pride one has in announcing the age.

"Good for you," several moms said in a chorus of support. Dena looked happy.

"Does anyone want to talk about how things are going?" Ilana lobbed the first question. "Now you're back at work?" Ilana asked a young and very fit mother of a small baby girl.

"I'm Jo and I'm back at work." The woman had translucent blue eyes, which were all the more startling against her brown skin. She held her daughter in her lap. "My daughter Violet is now four months and I was really scared I wouldn't be able to pump at work. I'm a police officer."

"So how's that going? You mentioned that you bought the car attachment so you could pump in your car." Ilana brought the group up to speed.

"It's going okay. I also have a battery power pack, the one for the Pump In Style, so I took the motor and everything out of its case so I could bring it with me. And I had to take some of the panels out of my vest as well. You know, when I felt full. God forbid anything ever happens. And if anyone ever found out." Jo motioned to the sky above. "The other day after work I came home and I couldn't wait to bring her to me." Jo hugged her daughter with both arms reaching around tight so there was a complete circle. "I love nursing her." I was in complete awe. "I was working a very big awards show. I was able to pump in the bathroom." I tried to imagine where she kept her milk for the rest of the evening. Did she keep her pump, motor, and all on her holster? I was too intimidated to ask for details, but I couldn't get enough of the story.

If Jo could fight crime and pump, then anyone could pump. I had gotten precious about the whole nursing and pumping thing. I went into a rage if Peter moved my pillows on the sofa. The story the nursing cop told brought it all into perspective for me.

Rachel told everyone about her recent trip to her in-laws. She had flown up to Canada a few days ahead of her husband. When he flew up to meet her he brought her breast pump. She related a funny story about her husband having to explain the breast pump to airport security. Everyone laughed.

I was about to go on and on about my progress when Dena interrupted.

"You know it's all just too much. I just can't do it." There was a tremble in her voice that kept me from turning around to look at her. "It hurts. I just can't bring him in."

"Well, why don't you latch him on so I can see how it's going?" Ilana got up from her seat and went by Dena's side. "How old is he again, you said ten days?"

"He's ten days old." As she brought her son in he began to wail with a high-pitched screech. Ilana made some adjustments and placed a "Brest Friend" pillow on Dena's lap. Ilana then slipped a little finger glove on her index finger and placed it into her baby's mouth.

"Why don't we try and cupfeed him formula to calm him down. Have you been cupfeeding him?"

"Only two ounces at a feeding because my husband thought he would want to nurse more if we fed him less. But when I ran into, I'm sorry what's your name again?"

"Lisa," I answered.

"When I ran into Lisa yesterday she said her daughter would take as much as five ounces." Rule number one: unless your husband is a certified lactation consultant or has successfully latched the baby on to his own nipple seek professional help.

"You know, let's give him as much as he'll take," Ilana suggested. The baby drank several ounces, finishing one cylinder. They opened another.

"If you want we could set up an appointment." Ilana handed Dena her card. "Do you have a pump? A pump can often stimulate milk production."

"I have the little one with the battery. A friend lent it to me."

107

"We don't really recommend that one. There are other pumps that are gentler. Also, you'll get more milk if you double pump."

I empathized with Dena. Nursing had made me cry on several occasions, but in private. I never wanted to cry at the group. I was too vulnerable as it was. When others teared up I felt emotional by proxy.

Dena was in a safe place surrounded by supportive moms. "You need to take it one feeding at a time," Jo offered Dena.

Rachel told Dena about her first three weeks nursing her daughter. "I knew she was drinking because I could hear her swallow, but I was in such pain."

"Lots of mothers have trouble in the beginning," the mother of two told her.

"It's really amazing you're even here. I am so impressed." Stephanie used the same line she gave me at the previous meeting.

Ilana and Dena continued to feed the baby more formula. He was hungry, very hungry. Once he seemed satiated they tried to latch him on, but he soon fell asleep.

By then I had successfully fed Sophie on my left breast, had burped her without a drop of spit up, and was about to latch her on my right breast when Ilana stopped me.

"Your nipples look an angry red. Let me look in her mouth." Since Sophie had already had some milk she wasn't quite as frantic. Ilana picked her up and looked at her tongue. "It's a little white in there, though it could just be milk."

"You think my nipples look red?" I pointed over to Rachel and said, "My nipples look like hers."

"That's because when she delatches she turns her head and pulls the nipple with her." Rachel demonstrated. She turned her head imitating her young daughter's pull on her breast. "How old?" Rachel asked me. "How old?" is the official mommy friend pick-up line in case you need one.

"She's one month old today."

108

"Lots of hair."

"Yeah, you know it hasn't fallen out yet." I had been told several times that Sophie's hair would fall out, which it had yet to do.

"And yours?"

"She's three months." Her daughter looked huge compared to my Sophie. And likewise my Sophie looked huge compared to Dena's newborn.

"It could be thrush." Ilana looked again in Sophie's mouth and then at my nipple.

"Thrush? What's that?" I had never heard of the term thrush. Again, a little reading of a good breast-feeding book would have gone a long way.

"It's a yeast infection."

"Wait, you can get a yeast infection on your nipple?"

"You know I had one with the first one and here I am with it again this time around," the mother of two called over to me. "I gave up on wearing a bra, I just leak and leak, it works better for me to not wear one. It lets air get to them." She was a large woman who wore a large loose-fitting denim shirt. Now, her breasts were *long*.

"What?" I knew the mother of two was trying to be supportive, but I was too appalled to take in what she was telling me. I couldn't believe that on top of the flat nipples, the engorgement, the freak nursing injury, and my wrist splint, I might have a yeast infection on my nipples.

I know I should have thanked my lucky stars that I was an over-producer, and of all the problems to have that was a good one, but I was beginning to feel like the Job of nursing.

"I think they're red because she has a very strong suck. See, I still need to support my breast just so or I get a pinch." I motioned with my hands the way I still needed to cup my fingers in a C shape in order to nurse Sophie pain free. I felt the need to make a statement. "I want everyone to know that I'm a very clean person."

"It doesn't have to do with that," the mother of two told me. I would much rather have burst into tears than have everyone in the room think I had thrush.

"Women get thrush all the time. Sometimes we're just susceptible to it. You should check with your doctor, it may *not* be thrush. It may be a sign that she's still pinching. Are you still feeling pain when she's nursing?" Ilana asked.

"Not really, sometimes, but I delatch her right away. I want everyone to know I don't have a yeast infection, so I am not sure it's thrush." I wanted to set the record straight on what yeast infections I could possibly have.

"One isn't connected to the other," the woman with two kids explained.

I wanted to say, "Hey you over there, that's enough." Here I was so hungry for new friends and I found myself being a snob. And there was a mother who wanted to offer me words of support and advice but I didn't want her words. I had felt the sting of being invisible to the mothers in my neighborhood, the ones with older children. I understood the mom hierarchy in this way: a new mom was a freshman, mothers with toddlers were sophomores, mothers who had one baby and another on the way were juniors, and mothers of two were seniors. In the end I felt most comfortable with other freshman, like Rachel, the mom with the red nipples. We already had something in common. As for the woman who went without a bra, leaking and everything, I just didn't think we were really clicking on the mommy level.

Around two-thirty the group cleared out. Dena and Ilana continued to work together. I left the meeting with Rachel.

"Your daughter's the first Sophie I've met." I was so naïve.

"Yeah, wasn't that wild how there were three Sophies at the group? Lisa, I'm telling you, in three months it is going to be so easy, she'll hold her head up. You'll pack the diaper bag with one arm while you've got her on your hip with the other." I loved that she remembered my name.

"I couldn't believe that police officer. She was so inspiring."

"Last time I was here, she told us about how she had to hang cloth diapers in her squad car so she could pump."

"Wow. I don't have thrush and I would never go without a bra, not even at night. I leak so much I still need the bra to keep my pads in place."

"I used to leak all the time. Now it's only in the morning."

"I told Ilana I didn't want to come to the group because I thought it was going to be all these crazy Nursing Nazi's. Now I can't tell you how much I looked forward to the group."

"I had Sophie in the dead of winter, I was stuck inside all the time. Now I notice I'm much happier if I go to the group."

"Last meeting there was a woman with a seven-month-old, who nursed using those tubes. I remember thinking if she can nurse a seven-month-old with tubes, then I can nurse my daughter through all my problems."

"I think I met her. She was at my first meeting. You know what I thought? I thought what have I gotten myself into?" I laughed at Rachel's comment a little harder than I should have, but she spoke my language.

"I was so surprised when that woman broke down. I ran into her and her husband yesterday. He told me their son was latching on great. And I met her for the first time a week and a half ago. Gave her my number, told her I knew an amazing lactation consultant, the group, the whole bit. She never called."

"Yeah, that was sad."

"I don't get it. If she was having trouble why didn't she get help?"

"You know I have a friend and she was going to breast-feed exclusively for a year, blah, blah, blah. She wouldn't hire a lactation consultant, too much money. Guess what? Not nursing at all."

"I couldn't get over how much help I needed. You know I had to have six or seven visits. It was pathetic."

"I didn't get help until Sophie was three weeks old. Like I said, I knew she was drinking and I counted diapers. But I was so sore." Rachel grabbed her chest as though it was still sore.

"What breast pads have you been using?" I asked.

Rachel recommended the Johnson and Johnson brand. "I like them because they have an indentation for the nipple." We compared notes on our gear. We talked pumps, bras, and pillows.

It was freshman orientation and I had found my buddy.

Chapter 9

Red Angry Nipples

I WAS HORRIFIED that my new friends at the group knew all about the alleged thrush condition of my nipples. I called Suzanne the moment I got home, despite the fact that Sophie was eager to nurse again and I couldn't use a pacifier. We had stopped using it several days before believing it may have contributed to the pinch. Sophie was not happy. Only nursing would soothe her to sleep, but this time she would have to wait.

It hadn't occurred to me that my midwife would go on vacation, but that's where she was. She wouldn't be back until the following week. Her receptionist had always been helpful, and without missing a beat she assured me I would be in good hands with the doctor on call. My midwife's backup was a male OB/GYN. The receptionist took my name and number and told me the doctor would have to call me back. Since I had her on the phone, I made the first available appointment with Suzanne for the following week.

I nursed Sophie to sleep and transferred her to her crib. I was getting good at moving her undisturbed. With her sleeping I was able to work the phones. My next call was to Sophie's pediatrician. He wasn't concerned in the least. He told me thrush was common, and there was no need to bring Sophie into the office. He told me I could use the over-the-counter antifungal gentian violet.

"Dab the inside of her mouth with the gentian violet with a Q-tip. Just a little, you only need a little. Keep doing that, and at her next checkup we'll take a look." The pediatrician had also recommended dabbing gentian violet on my breasts as well. He was a little curt with me when I suggested I get something a little stronger and assured me again the gentian violet would work. I had never heard of gentian violet. Turns out none of the big chain pharmacies had heard of it either. I couldn't find anyone local that carried the magic potion. But that was what the pediatrician recommended. Peter and I had some misgivings about our pediatrician being in the city as opposed to Brooklyn. We had both wanted to find someone local who was within running distance. I decided that once I took care of the thrush situation I would look into finding another pediatrician. He was great at the hospital, but I was less thrilled with his phone manners.

In the meantime I made a call to one of my few friends with children. "Guess what?" I took a breath before I revealed my secret, "I think I have thrush."

"You have thrush!" she exclaimed. "My neighbor has thrush, too. She's over right now." She laughed. I guess it was going around. I could hear her friend laugh as well. "I had it, too. You just need to get that ointment. You put it in the baby's mouth and on your breast and it'll clear up soon enough."

"Do you mean gentian violet?"

"Gentian what? Never heard of that. It was some cream or ointment. I got a prescription from my doctor."

"I never heard of thrush before."

"Oh Lisa, it's *in* all the books."

"How did you know it was thrush?"

114

"After I nursed her, I thought, what a good eater, because she had all this milk in her mouth. It looked a little like cottage cheese and I brushed it away and then I saw blood."

"Is there anything else?" I said half joking. "Is there anything else I should be on the lookout for?"

"Just watch out for that really bad diaper rash. It looks like someone put the baby on a burner. All the Balmex in the world won't clear that up. It's yeast. You need to put cream on it, the kind they use for athlete's foot."

"Wait, you put athlete's foot cream on her bottom?"

"Yeah, it takes care of it right away."

"Thanks for the info. We'll have to get together soon."

"Right, right," she said. Somehow I knew we wouldn't have our senior-freshman outing anytime soon.

An hour after I spoke with my friend, the doctor called. He prescribed Diflucan, which is a pill that treats yeast systemically.

"Could I just get a prescription for the cream? I'm not even sure if I have thrush, so I don't know if I really need to take something orally."

Ilana had suggested seeing my doctor or midwife to find out if what I had was the result of thrush or a pinch. To be fair I could have gone in for an appointment but I didn't feel comfortable with a male doctor examining my nipples. Aside from my dentist and ophthalmologist all of my doctors were female. That was the dynamic I preferred.

I had hoped for the ointment my friend told me about. That seemed simple enough. He explained that if it was indeed thrush, the cream or ointment wasn't always effective. I would end up taking the pill anyway. There was no point arguing, he was not going to prescribe the cream. I had him call in the prescription anyway.

"If you want a second opinion, call the birthing center." He even gave me the number.

After I hung up I called the birthing center. I spoke with their lactation consultant who was on call. She reiterated what the doctor told me. As is often the case with thrush, a topical cream doesn't always knock out the yeast, so they prescribed Diflucan as well. She went on to tell me that the medication was considered safe for nursing mothers. That was part of the reason I was reluctant to take another pill. Since Sophie was born I had taken untold amounts of Motrin, stool softeners (you may need a few of those that first week after delivery), and the antibiotics I was given in the hospital because I had tested positive for group B strep. Here I was nursing for the health benefits and God knows what was being passed on through my breast milk.

I called Ilana. I told her that my midwife was out of town for the week and that the doctor on call prescribed the pill. "Why such big guns?" Ilana asked. She went on to tell me that I really needed to get examined in person, and if I could wait until next week to see the midwife that might be best. But I was impatient, I feared that if it was the early stages of thrush it was going to get worse and cause me more problems with nursing.

"What's the name of the cream women use?" I asked.

"I believe some women treat it with the ointment Nystatin. I believe there are several kinds you could use." As Ilana spoke I scribbled the word Nystatin in the back of my phone book.

"I'll tell you what happens."

I hung up and called Peter at work. He listened to the whole red angry nipples story. I told him about some purple liquid called gentian violet, about my conversation with the doctor, and the fact that all I had by the end of that afternoon was a prescription for a pill.

Peter said he would make a few calls for gentian violet. Next he suggested that I call his father. My father-in-law was a pulmonary specialist. He had been listed for years as one of the best doctors in New York by *New York* magazine and had been nationally recognized as well.

"He's a doctor and could always write you a prescription." I had thought about calling his father, but since it involved me discussing my nipples I decided against it. If I kept it vague, it didn't seem like such a bad idea.

"How's your wrist?" Peter asked. With all the commotion about my nipples I almost forgot about my nursing injury.

"It's feeling better. Thanks, I love you."

"I love you, too." Peter hung up. If he wasn't Jewish I would have suspected that he was vying to be canonized.

I took a deep breath and called my father-in-law. He wasn't in his office, so I asked his secretary to page him.

"Hi, dear."

"Listen I need you to write a prescription for an anti-fungal cream, I think it's called Nystatin." I explained how my midwife was out of town, that my lactation consultant thought both Sophie and I had thrush, and that Sophie's pediatrician had prescribed gentian violet.

"Gentian violet! I haven't heard about that in years," my father-in-law said.

"Well that's what her doctor suggested."

"So it's in her mouth?"

"I think so, it doesn't look like cottage cheese, there's a little white on her tongue. But I was hoping to just start with the cream, otherwise I'm going to dab gentian violet in her mouth. And I'm supposed to dab it on me as well. You know if the baby gets thrush in her mouth, then the mother has it as well."

"I'm not sure that's going to do anything. I don't do things over the phone. When you come out to the Island, I'll take a look. I saw tons of thrush when I was in the service." My father-in-law had been an officer during the Vietnam War working at an army hospital outside Philadelphia. I had no idea thrush was so common. Were soldiers getting it from dirty shirts? I couldn't imagine how all those soldiers in got thrush on their nipples. Maybe they just had it in their mouths? It made no sense, but I had more pressing issues to discuss.

"You'll take a look at her?"

"I'll take a look at both of you." He tried to be reassuring, but I found it appalling that he wanted to examine me as well.

"You know I really don't feel comfortable about that. Couldn't you just take my word and prescribe some cream? I'd even take a sample if you have that."

"Would you stop? I'll see you later tonight. Don't worry. I've seen it hundreds of times."

"I really don't feel comfortable, I think it would be very awkward. I could give you the number of my pharmacy and you could just call it in?"

"I'll see you later tonight. After I take a look I will feel more comfortable prescribing something. Bye, hon." And with those words my father-in-law hung up.

I sat straight up on our couch. Did I just hear my father-in-law right? He wanted to examine my breasts, more specifically my nipples? The father of my husband wanted me to show him my red angry nipples. How could this be? I didn't feel comfortable about nursing in front of him, much less showing him my nipples up close and personal.

How did I get to this point? I called Peter again.

"Peter, you're not going to believe this. Your dad wants to examine my nipples to see if I have thrush." I knew Peter would be just as mortified as I was.

"Well, he is a doctor." Wrong answer.

"Let me get this straight, you want me to show your dad my nipples?"

"Well, if you don't feel comfortable you should just tell him."

"I did tell him. He said he doesn't like prescribing things over the phone." The fact that my husband didn't respond with shock was a problem. Peter had been a witness to my nursing drama for weeks. He no longer knew what was right, what was gross, or most of all what to say to me.

I decided to call my father-in-law back. I had him paged again.

"Hi, Harry. Look, I will let you look at Sophie's mouth, but I just don't feel comfortable with you examining me. Okay? So if it looks like Sophie has thrush, then you'll prescribe the cream?"

"Would you stop, it'll take a second. Look I just spoke with our lactation consultant here at the hospital, she suggested boiling all the parts to your breast pump. You need to be very careful." Until that moment it never occurred to me that I should sterilize the parts to my breast pump. I had rinsed them occasionally, but sometimes I had pumped, left the pump there and several hours later, pumped again. What was wrong with me, why hadn't I been treating the pumps in a more sanitary fashion? Make sure you sterilize your pump parts according to the manufacturer's directions. Some of the parts can go in the top rack of the dishwasher.

"Ewww . . . will do." The conversation was embarrassing. "Well, I just can't do it." I was holding firm.

In my mind the scene from a bad movie was playing. I would be sitting on an ottoman. Next to me was my husband. My father-in-law would have some doctor tool, like a magnifying glass. "Now why don't we see those red angry nipples?" he would say.

"I don't understand the problem." My father-in-law was miffed. You could hear it in his voice.

"The problem? You don't understand the problem? You don't understand why looking at my nipples would make me uncomfortable?"

"Your nipples?" He was quiet for a moment.

"Harry?" I wasn't sure if he was still on the other end.

"I thought we were talking about your mouth."

"My mouth? How would I get thrush in my mouth?"

"That's what I didn't understand." Harry was exasperated.

"I thought you wanted to look at my nipples."

"Nope." Again there was a silence from his end. Then he said, "Okay, that's the end of this conversation."

"I guess so." I should have pursued the prescription anyway, but I just wanted to get off the phone.

"See you later tonight, around seven?" he said, breaking what was a long pause.

"Sounds good." It was all just a misunderstanding, a *Who's On First* except with nipples and mouths.

Early that evening Peter returned home with several small bottles of gentian violet. He found them at a family owned pharmacy and, to be on the safe side, bought up their stock. They were cheap and Peter had no idea how much we needed.

I took a swab and dipped just the tip of it into the gentian violet, covering an area no larger than a pea. I then put the swab into Sophie's mouth and lightly dabbed the sides of her cheeks. Before I could pull it out, she sucked on it. Just like that her mouth, her lips, even her chin was stained a deep dark purple. My beautiful darling had an angry purple mouth, stained just in time for the big visit with the family later that night. Peter walked into the bedroom and looked down at Sophie who was still on the changing table.

"Is that what you were supposed to do?"

"I think I used too much."

"Look at her." Peter picked Sophie up. She was dressed in one of her fancier outfits, which was quickly being stained by purple drool.

"Let's just get out of here and on the road," I told him.

"Who's got a purple mouth?" Peter said to Sophie. "Who's got a purple mouth? You do." I know I wouldn't have been that calm if he had made her all purple. Right before we left I went into the bathroom and locked the door. I took out another swab, dipped it into gentian violet and dabbed it on my nipples. Even if it didn't do anything, I figured purple was better than red.

WE SPENT that weekend with Peter's folks. I don't think I looked my father-in-law in the eye the entire time. We have boxes and boxes of photos from Sophie's first year, but none from that weekend. Sophie looked like she had her lips tattooed purple. And it took days for the gentian violet to fade. But it did. And of course we never applied it again. She spit up purple that whole night and we had only applied it once. Her crib, her bumper, her clothes were all stained purple.

As Peter put it, "I'd rather have her have thrush than stain everything we own purple."

The following Monday I switched Sophie to a local pediatrician just a few blocks from our home. He examined her mouth and told me she didn't have thrush.

MONTHS LATER I had the nerve to ask my father-in-law a question that had bothered me since our first bit of confusion with the thrush.

"What did you mean when you told me you saw a lot of thrush in the service? Was it common for GI's to get it in their mouths?" I asked him.

"What I said was I saw a lot of thrush on service, meaning on the hospital service, not in the service. In pulmonary we see oral thrush most commonly in patients with weakened immune systems or those who use orally inhaled steroids, like those used by asthmatics." And later we were able to laugh about the whole thing, but that took nearly a year to achieve.

As for my possible thrush, a week later I finally saw Suzanne. She told me that no, I didn't have thrush. What I did have was a rough nursling. There was still a pinch. The latch still wasn't right.

121

Chapter 10

The "Vacation"

BY LATE SPRING evening strolls became our nightly ritual. Peter would come home, change his clothes, and out we went. Most nights we brought Halley along. Between our dog and Sophie's SUV we were a large bulky presence and must have annoyed all who crossed our path.

We noticed a couple walking toward us. They had that new-parent look, which could best be described as disheveled, but unlike us they were traveling light. The father had their baby in the carrier.

"Hi there, how do you like that thing?" I asked, pointing to their carrier.

"I love it." Their baby appeared to be a few weeks younger than Sophie.

"You have a new one as well," the father said. He was beaming. Perhaps that's the look of a new parent, disheveled and beaming. We peeked at theirs and they peeked at ours. Both were asleep.

"Are you nursing?" I tried my best to sound cool.

She said "Yes."

"How's it going?"

"I think it's going okay." She looked a tad bewildered by my question.

"You know there's a breast-feeding support group that meets every other Wednesday. Lots of new moms are there. It's free and a lactation consultant runs it. It's on the maternity floor of the hospital down the block. It's meeting this coming Wednesday if you're interested. Boy or girl?" I took a second look at her baby and tried not to sound weird.

"This is Oscar, he's four weeks old."

"This is Sophie, almost six weeks, and I'm Lisa and that's Peter," I said, pointing in Peter's direction.

"I'm Jamie and this is Robert. You know, I just might check it out."

"I'll be there," I told her. Both she and her husband thanked us and waved good-bye.

"I think you freaked her out," Peter said once they were out of earshot. I could tell he was uncomfortable with my new way with strangers.

"No, I thought she seemed genuinely interested. I wouldn't be surprised if she showed up."

Before I had Sophie I never would have strode up to strangers and pushed a support group, now I found it difficult not to. We passed another couple that night. As we drew closer Peter begged, "Oh no, please don't." So for Peter's sake we said hello and walked on by.

THAT WEDNESDAY I arrived early at the group. Several moms were there and Laura, not Ilana, was leading the meeting. The mom I had recruited from the street was there, too. The woman pointed at me and said, "She's the one who told me about the meeting."

"You're Oscar's mom, right?" I was reminded of my early days with Halley at the dog run. I always knew the name of the dog, not the owner.

"Yes, is it Lisa?"

"Yes, and your name? I'm sorry I forgot."

"Jamie."

"So glad you made it." The fact that Jamie came to that meeting gave me a false sense of the power of my suggestions. I remember thinking, "See, if they know about it they will come." Jamie wouldn't be the last woman I approached about the group. There would be others and in the end several would take down the information and make it to the meeting. At least a half dozen showed up over time, but usually women looked at me as though I had offered to sell them the leftovers from my fridge.

I was happy to see Rachel there as well. Rachel leaned over to me and said, "I thought it was you. She told us a woman stopped her on the street." I took it as a compliment. I looked around the room again. Dena, the new mom I had met several weeks before, was absent.

I hadn't seen Laura since my first appointment and I told her all about my progress: "It's going well, she's almost exclusively on breast milk. She's just taking an ounce or two of formula per day."

The room was filling up and once things settled down I turned to Laura. "Could I make an announcement?"

"Of course." Maybe she thought I was selling cookies.

I stood up. "Hi everyone, I just have a little announcement to make. Last time at the meeting Ilana thought I might have thrush and I just wanted to let everyone know that I don't have thrush. Not that there's anything wrong with that. I know lots of women who have had it. But I don't." I held Sophie up Exhibit A style. "I went to the doctor and my daughter has a very rough suck. We still need to work on the latch. That's all." I took my seat.

"Okay," Laura said. I wasn't looking for applause. I was simply setting the record straight.

Another new mom strolled into the group.

"I know you," Jamie said to the woman. "We were in prenatal yoga."

"Oh right, how's it going?"

"I ended up having a C-section and this is Oscar. He was over nine pounds." The petite Jamie held up her giant newborn. The other new mom's name was Norma. She stood at over six feet tall and was enormous.

"This is Lilly. She was nine pounds, four ounces."

"Did you end up having a C-section?" Jamie asked.

"No, by the time I got to the hospital I was fully dilated, so I just pushed. It was too late for drugs," Norma said with pride.

That must have been some yoga class.

"I had a pretty bad rectal tear," she explained. There was a lot of sharing in that group. Then Norma made a mini announcement of her own. "Also, I gained over sixty pounds. I had the worst case of edema." What new mom couldn't relate? We were all walking disclaimers. "I latched her on with you yesterday, it went great," Norma told Laura. "Then you left and I haven't latched her on since."

"Doesn't it always go better when they're in the room?" I added.

"I once had a mother who recorded my voice and instruction to latch her baby on and she would play it when she nursed. She said it always helped." Then Laura turned to Norma. "Let's see what's going on." I wish I had thought of recording her voice after our first session. It was a great idea and if you can, I recommend doing it. I'm sure it would have helped me in my early weeks.

When Laura was through working with the new mom and her baby girl, she came over to me.

I was fussing around with Sophie's cloth diaper, but she was larger now and it was difficult to wrap her up.

"Why don't you try and bring her in without the diaper," Laura pulled the cloth away. Sophie no longer flailed about. I had been so used to the ritual that I hadn't noticed. For the first time without the cloth diaper I brought her in with one big swoosh and on she went. It was a good latch right away.

"So when are you giving her formula?"

"Only at night when we run out of breast milk."

"Do you think you could latch her on then?"

"I could try, is formula bad?"

"No, many mothers need to supplement with formula. But there are no benefits with formula, and there are health benefits with breast milk. When you supplement, when you introduce formula or solids to their intake it cuts into the benefits of breast milk. So if you are pumping enough to give her only breast milk, then that is what you want to try and do. Or instead of pumping, experiment and see if you can latch her on at the night feeding. Most mothers have trouble with the night feeding, but see if you can."

"I haven't attempted that in a while, I tend to want to pump because I'm afraid of getting a pinch."

"Well, keep doing what you're doing. It sounds good, but if you can, when you feel up to it, try to latch her on instead."

"How old is she?"

"Six weeks."

"Now six weeks is another growth spurt, so she'll be getting your supply up and will nurse more than usual," Laura said. I had been told about the three-week, six-week, and three-month growth spurts. They still caught me off guard.

"She already cluster feeds in the evenings."

"Good. Just keep offering." In the evenings Sophie would nurse often. It seemed nonsensical the way I would feed her and less than a half hour later she would want to nurse again. So I would offer and she would latch back on. And that's how it was during her growth spurts. I had survived the three-week growth spurt and I must have entered the six-week spurt the day before. I offered and offered and she just nursed and nursed. If I viewed each feeding as the method Sophie used to increase my supply then the feedings made sense. And that was exactly how Ilana and Laura taught me to view them. I had the confidence of Sophie's weight gain to know that indeed she was getting enough and never viewed her feedings as me being deficient of "not having enough milk," as I knew some women worried was the case.

The group's conversation turned to pumping plans, latches, tubes, and when to start cereal.

I walked out with Rachel and Jamie.

"I wish you were here last time, there was this amazing woman who was a cop," I told Jamie. I was disappointed Jo wasn't there. She was the closest thing to a nursing superhero as I would ever know.

"She was so inspiring, pumped on the job, the whole bit," Rachel added. "Carried the parts of her Pump In Style on her holster."

We walked on a bit farther then said our good-byes.

I SPENT the next day packing and nursing. We were taking the baby and dog to Newport, Rhode Island. Newport was the winter home of my favorite great aunt and I had visited it nearly every winter for the first eighteen years of my life. After she died I hadn't returned until a job brought me back the year before. I was filming a fund-raising video and had to interview several students at a nearby private school. Peter came along and we stayed at a small inn on the water, right near the famed Black Pearl restaurant. The best part was that they allowed dogs. I had worked both days, but we still had a memorable getaway.

When three episodes from my television series were programmed to screen at the Newport International Film Festival it was an excuse to go on our first family vacation. I made reservations last minute and saw it as fate that the inn we liked so much had a room available. It was the very same one we had stayed in the year before. After six weeks in the nether world of nursing troubles the festival was going to provide the perfect escape. I was excited to bring Sophie along and couldn't wait to show her off. She was all smiles by six weeks. And I would be able to make more contacts for my company, meet up with friends, and most of all, it was going to be romantic. Though not *too* romantic—it had only been six weeks since Sophie was born.

We were invited to several parties and my parents were going to meet us in Newport to babysit. Because Sophie was now old enough to take a bottle we could actually leave my parents with a bottle of breast milk. We were through with the messy cupfeedings. We had practiced with the bottle twice before and she drank away with no nipple confusion.

Baby and dog would share the back seat and my Medela Classic would be safely tucked in the trunk. If you travel with your pump, make sure you have all the parts packed as well. Several are small and easy to misplace, which was exactly what we had done the week before. Peter spent a panicked afternoon in Long Island and nearly fifty bucks buying a part. I, of course, feared getting engorged. I wasn't pumping like I did during Sophie's first few weeks, but I needed to know that if I felt full and had trouble latching Sophie on I *could* pump. So I checked every piece of equipment for the trip to Newport. Feeling adventurous, I also packed the BabyBjörn.

IT SHOULD have taken us about five hours to get to Newport, but with traffic as heavy as it was and the fact that I nursed Sophie in the parking lot of a Boston Market, the trip took seven. A brief word about nursing in a parking lot: avoid it if you can. An air-conditioned restaurant is far more comfortable and usually offers more privacy than the parking lot. Nursing in the car is never as discreet as you think. It would take a few more parking lots before I figured that out. And I know this goes without saying, but it is unwise to travel with a dog when you have a newborn. We had had the best time with Halley the year before. She loved running up and down Newport's Cliff Walk and was a great travel companion. But things had changed. After I pulled the tenth hair out of Sophie's mouth, I mentioned to Peter that perhaps we should have left Halley home.

By the time we arrived in Newport we were covered in an absurd amount of dog hair. My parents were waiting for us at the inn. We had just enough time to shower and change our clothes. Then I nursed Sophie. We had to assemble the co-sleeper, which we were using as a portable crib. Like the car seat, it took longer than expected. The frame of the crib had to be snapped together, which in the process pinched Peter's fingers giving him blood blisters. My father tried to help, which entailed several comments like, "You know you should write a letter to the company who made this and tell them what a piece of crap it is." Or, "You should take this back." Or, "In our day I think we used a box." I thought Peter was going to give up. He kept yanking up the sides of the crib with great force. Changing his technique, he pulled slowly. It clicked. At last we were off.

It was the first time we had left Sophie for an evening, and what better reason than a swanky party? It was a catered affair at a mansion on the water. There was even a celebrity sighting in the form of Lee Majors. He looked like he was having a good time. On the patio we met up with some friends. "See, having a baby doesn't really have to change your life," I told myself. I drank one white wine spritzer, which after our road trip tasted like nectar. It was to become my drink of choice while nursing. We stood with our friends out by the water and I talked briefly about the series, but all I thought about was

129

Sophie. She had entered a super cute stage and I found myself hugging and holding her all the time. I loved to talk to her in my high-pitched mommy voice. She would smile and respond to my coos. We could have stayed out later, but after two hours we were both eager to head home. We missed her.

When we returned to the room Sophie was happy. Ready to nurse, but happy. My parents had offered her the bottle, but she only took an ounce or so. "She's not crazy about that bottle. She mostly played with the nipple," my mom reported.

"She may not have been hungry," I told my mom, but any practice was good for her. We were using the bottles my lactation consultants had recommended, the Avent brand. The large silicone nipples were preferable for nursing babies because the wide surface area kept the baby from pinching tightly on the nipple. Other types such as the latex nipples for disposable bottles, give the baby a tiny nipple surface to suck. This, in turn, can create a pinch when the mother nurses.

We had remembered the room as spacious but with Sophie's crib, the dog, makeshift changing area, pumping station, and other baby paraphernalia, the room took on the claustrophobic feeling of a family youth hostel. One could barely get around the bed. We were visiting our old life with all the baggage of our new one.

SOPHIE WOKE up around four o'clock in the morning. It was early for her considering that she had made it all the way to six o'clock several times that week, but between the traveling and her growth spurt I was surprised she slept as long as she did. Usually I would have pumped while Peter gave Sophie breast milk or formula, but I was too tired. I had hit that moment when it was easier to nurse than to pump.

130

"Here give her to me, I'll nurse her," I told Peter as I strapped on my pillow.

"Are you sure?" Peter handed Sophie to me. I brought her in. The latch was good and she nursed. Peter didn't know it then, but he was free. No more night feedings for him. I would be the one feeding her from then on. She nursed until she fell asleep and I transferred her back into the crib. What had just happened was big. I thought, "Can't wait to tell the group about this. No more formula."

Our hope had been to go out for breakfast before the screening, which was at ten in the morning. But it took hours to get out of that tiny room. The morning was a primping and nursing extravaganza. My makeup was a little heavy for a June morning and my hair was blown out and curled. It was all a diversion. I hoped people wouldn't notice my weight. And since nothing fit, I wore a white polo and khaki pants. I would have worn a dress in my pre-baby days, but I couldn't wear a dress and nurse—not that any fit. There are some companies that specialized in nursing wear. One could buy swimsuits, shirts, and dresses all with pull-back panels that enable you to nurse. But I never saw anything that was my style. Most of the dresses were usually made out of rayon in loud prints, but that morning I regretted not having one.

We made it to the theater right at ten o'clock. We parked Sophie in the aisle and took the seats next to her in the back row of the theater. It was a completely different experience seeing the series blown up on the big screen. I watched the episodes from the series and halfway through Sophie woke up and I nursed her. I looked down at her, then up at the screen, then back at her. The audience responded well to the work. My parents were proud. It made the car ride and trouble all worth it.

We mingled a bit after the screening.

"You guys are too much, here with a six-week-old, how do you do it?" a friend asked. As pleased as I was with the screening, what

131

brought me my greatest source of joy that day was the fact that our little family didn't appear as disheveled as we felt.

"We just pack up and go. Nothing to it," I lied.

"Lisa, you amaze me, here with the baby, you didn't skip a beat," another friend said. We resembled a high-functioning couple with our "nothing's going to slow us down" motto. But it was all a charade.

ONCE EVERYONE cleared out of the theater we headed to lunch with my parents. Sophie was all smiles. My father shot off a roll of film. There's even a photo of me. It was shot from behind, taken while I was nursing Sophie. That's right: I nursed Sophie in a restaurant with the pillow around my waist. All you can see from the photo is my back, the side of my face, the pillow's Velcro belt, and Sophie's tiny feet sticking out. I was most likely saying something like, "Dad, please don't take a picture." But he did. The other photos are of Sophie. She was so cute in her blue dress with its intricate smocking. Even if *you* can't dress well, your baby can. My parents were in grandparents' heaven. If they could have stayed longer they would have, but they had another engagement.

Once they left we went back to the room for a nap. We had the festival schedule and assumed we would head out to another screening a few hours later. Somehow between the nap and Sophie's nursing we were unable to get out of our hotel room for nine hours. I kept looking at the festival schedule. "Maybe we could make the next screening," I'd tell Peter. I would fix my hair, nurse, change my clothes, and so on. By the time we got it together to leave it was dark out.

Newport gets crowded in the summer, and down by the water at night it gets very crowded. The stroller didn't seem like a good idea. It was time to try the baby carrier. Peter put on the carrier and I slid

132

Sophie down into it. Though it was June, it was a cool evening with a bit of a breeze, so Sophie wore a hat and I wrapped a receiving blanket around her as well.

We headed out to the festival's clambake. Our pace was slow and deliberate. We saw lots of college guys on the prowl and several bachelorette parties. They were easy to spot because someone was always wearing a small faux veil. One drunken kid even yelled to a bride-to-be, "Hey you're too fat to marry." I was incensed. Pre-baby I would have yelled back at the jerk, but now I was with precious cargo and felt too vulnerable to mix it up. Maybe it was because Sophie was so young, or because she was in the baby carrier, but the streets of Newport, Rhode Island, seemed scary that night.

"Let's get going," I told Peter.

"Do you think she's breathing?" he said. We stopped. Sophie was asleep and her face was mashed against Peter's chest. I turned her head so it was facing out to the side and gave her a gentle poke until she moved.

"She's breathing." We would play that game several more times that night.

Though the clambake was only a few blocks away, it felt like a long walk. Peter tried to take some food but didn't attempt sitting down, not with Sophie in the carrier.

"You look tense," someone said to him.

"I am," he said. That first test-drive with the baby carrier gave Peter a backache for days, not because Sophie was heavy, but because he was so stiff.

We met up with friends from New York and stood around discussing the festival, the screening, and, of course, our six-week-old. Another woman walked over to our group. She was from Boston and was at the festival with her partner. She looked very pregnant.

"You must be due any day," I told her after we made our initial introductions.

"Just five months along. I'm huge right?"

"Wow, that's some big baby." Every woman carries differently.

"Are you planning to nurse?" There I was again, right away asking the nursing question.

"Yes."

"I hope you get professional help."

"What do you mean?"

"Nursing isn't something you're born knowing how to do." I tried not to sound crazy, but the very sight of pregnant women did something to me. "I can help them," played in my mind. She was a good listener, but since I didn't know her well, I couldn't tell if her expression was fear, panic, or that she simply thought I was a nut. "It's not this thing that you instinctively know how to do. I had to have seven separate visits with a lactation consultant to get it right. I was bruised. I bled. I could have avoided all of it had I just been a little more educated."

"Wait, what do you mean, I thought I would just pop the baby on." She motioned with her arms, holding a pretend baby, and gestured lifting the head of the baby into her chest, not unlike the scene from *The Blue Lagoon*.

"I thought that, too, but there is a skill to getting the right latch. Also," I moved in close to whisper, "I had flat nipples." I looked around me to make sure no one else was listening. "And guess what? I never knew I had flat nipples. And you need a lactation consultant because you may not know until the twentieth feeding that you're doing it wrong, and by then you're in pain."

"Wow, this reminds me of that conversation I had during school recess when my girlfriend told me what intercourse really was."

"You know it's like that, women don't talk about it." I hadn't really articulated before what I felt about nursing and its current place in the smart gal's rumor culture. It was my moment of yelling from the rooftops, "Hey ladies, nursing is a skill, an art that can take some practice." Peter came over to us.

"I think we should head back before she wakes up," Peter said. He was right. It was getting windy and I knew I wouldn't feel comfortable nursing there at the clambake.

"Hope I didn't scare you."

"No, I need to know this stuff," she said.

"Good luck," I told her. We left the party and headed back to our room.

After nursing Sophie I placed her back in her crib. I figured she would be up again in a few hours and was shocked when we all woke up around seven-thirty in the morning. It was the best night's sleep we had gotten since Sophie was born. Vive la difference, we all felt as though we had a new lease on life. Peter ran out for coffee and scones and we packed up in a little under an hour. We triple-checked the room to be sure we had all our crap and I made sure we had our ticket stubs from my screening. I planned to use them in Sophie's baby book.

WE KNEW we had a long ride home, but since we had an early start we decided for old time's sake to take the baby and dog to Newport's Cliff Walk before we left town. The Cliff Walk is just that, a trail that takes you along the cliff overlooking the water on one side and the huge summer "cottages" on the other. It was the quintessential summer morning, sunny and clear. Once again we snapped Sophie into the BabyBjörn.

Peter and I gave each other a knowing smile. Ah . . . we were living the fantasy. The day before had just been a fluke, one of those rough days. Now things were just like before, only better. We headed down the walk. Peter had Sophie and I had Halley on her leash. We took in the stunning views and made good time walking nearly to the end of the trail. We hadn't listened to the weather and that morning

135

didn't feel particularly hot. But when we were about four block lengths from the end of the trail, we started feeling the heat.

"How's she doing?"

Peter looked down at her. "I can't tell if she's sweating or if that's me."

"She looks hot," I said. I couldn't tell if Sophie was in a deep sleep or had succumbed to the heat.

"Did that carrier have a warning on it about hot days?" Peter asked.

"I'm not sure."

"Maybe we should turn around. It's really hot."

"Let's go back to the car." We turned around and picked up our pace. It was difficult to tell if we were hot because we had walked so much, or if the temperature did spike up.

"Maybe you should take her out of that thing," I told Peter.

"Should I just carry her?"

I hadn't even brought sunscreen or a hat. What were we thinking? We stopped and took Sophie out of the carrier. I had a cloth diaper with me so I draped that over her. Peter held her the way you would hold a hot casserole. Halley was leashed and walking right at my side. I didn't even notice the family with a dog coming toward us, why would I? We considered Halley a dog's dog. For whatever reason, maybe Halley thought Sophie was injured, or she was being protective, or she was no longer a dog's dog. Halley went for the other dog. She lurched forward pulling me with her and growled in *Cujo*-like ways. I yanked all eighty hairy pounds of her and walked ahead pulling her with me. I believe there was shrieking and yelling involved. It was one of those ugly moments. What stressed me out more was that we had at least a fifteen-minute walk to go. There would be other dogs.

It must have been in the nineties, much hotter than the night before or even that morning. The whole way I kept looking back at

136

Peter and Sophie. "How's she doing?" I must have asked a dozen times. I knew babies were susceptible to heatstroke. Every summer there seemed to be several tragic incidents involving infants and parked cars. I knew the temperature on the walk was nowhere near that kind of heat. There were two other dog incidents but I was prepared. I pulled on Halley's collar and told her to heel. I didn't have the strength in my wrists that I needed, but somehow I managed.

"I can't wait to get back to the car," Peter called ahead to me. I had to remind myself to breathe. I was holding my breath and didn't even realize it.

Our car was parked down the hill from the trailhead. It was sitting there in the sun. Peter handed Sophie to me, she felt hot but everything felt hot. He started the car and blasted the air conditioner. I sat there in the front seat with Sophie on my lap. I was too hot to nurse and she seemed groggy. It took several minutes before the car became comfortably cool.

"That was a close one," Peter said.

"Do you think she's okay?"

"She looks okay." She was breathing, her lips weren't dry and chapped—a good sign. It could have been the heat that conked her out or she might have been sleeping off that bender of growth spurt, either way she looked fine. And I was able to wake her up long enough to nurse. I didn't want to drive on until I knew she had more to drink. Had we stayed out longer, had we kept her in the carrier, any of those things could have caused dehydration or worse.

Our lives weren't the same. We wanted to go on walks in the midday heat, we wanted to travel with our dog, and go out to parties. We could still do all of that, but in slow motion, and with long pauses. We had new lives. We just didn't know how they worked yet.

WHEN WE RETURNED to Brooklyn there was a message on our machine. "Not sure if this is the right Lisa Shapiro, but several of us from the group are getting together to meet in the park this Friday at twelve-thirty, and since there is no meeting at the hospital this Wednesday we are going to meet at the park at twelve-thirty as well. So if you're around, hope you can make it. Beep." I was sorry I had missed the Friday soiree; we had already left for the film festival. But I couldn't wait for Wednesday.

WEDNESDAY was another perfect June day. I spotted Rachel when I arrived at the park. Jamie strolled in, as did Norma. I met Suzy, along with her baby girl. Finally we all took our seats along a row of benches in the shade. The new moms kept coming. Within a half hour there were seven of us. I went over the pitfalls of going on "vacation" with your newborn. Suzy told everyone her birth story, which included an ambulance and a delivery in triage.

Word had spread of the new mothers' group and several more moms came by and took their seats. There was talk about nannies and going back to work. Several commented on how they disliked a popular nursing pillow and were converts to the "Brest Friend." One woman touted her own rapid weight loss. Aside from her, I thought all of the women to be friendly, supportive, and funny.

There was nowhere on earth I would have rather been than there on those benches on that June day. I didn't want to be at a posh film festival, not flying off to some location for a shoot, not shopping in Midtown. I just wanted to sit with my new friends in the park and nurse the afternoon away.

Part Two

THE MOMENT she had laid the child to the breast both became perfectly calm.

ISAK DINESEN
Ehrengard

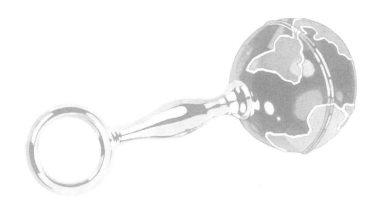

Chapter 11

It Gets Easier

BY MID-SUMMER I finally had gotten around to some reading. *The Nursing Mother's Companion* by Kathleen Huggins described the first two months of nursing as the "Learning Period." The second stage was called the "Reward Period," which went from two months to six months. Sophie was two months old and I was eager for that reward period to kick in, but it hadn't yet. I couldn't get out of the learning period, or more appropriately the survival period. Yes, Sophie cooed, smiled, and giggled. I loved being with her and hated leaving her when I had to. I had the habit of running my fingers through her black curls. We had all those tender *Baby Mine* moments, but when it came to nursing I was surviving each feeding. I still wore my wrist splint but was rid of most of my nursing contraptions and the process had been streamlined. Some feedings went well, but most were a mixed bag of slight pinching, sweating, and performance anxiety. For the last few weeks I was growing discouraged that I would ever achieve easy nursing.

SOCIALLY when I had come across other new moms, at work functions, at picnics, at parties, the conversation turned to breast-feeding. What I was always looking for was this. "When did you hit the reward period?"

One woman I met at a friend's birthday picnic told me one of the more horrifying nursing stories. She told me about the enormous amounts of blood her son would spit up after he nursed.

"It hurt so much, I was in pain the whole time," she confided.

"Did you get a lactation consultant?"

"No, but the person who rented me the pump gave me some instruction."

"Are you still nursing?"

"No, as soon as he turned four months, I stopped, which was a little silly because it had just gotten easy at that point. But four months was my goal, so I stopped."

"Four months is my goal," I told her.

"Good luck."

I was amazed that someone could be in that much pain for that long and not seek help. What disturbed me most about her experience was that she quit right when she had entered the reward period. I decided that if I hadn't hit the reward period by my fourth month I would wean Sophie. But if nursing became easy and I hit that magical reward period before she turned four months, then I would keep on nursing.

PETER HAD TO take a four-day trip out to the West Coast so I knew I was in for a long four days. I enlisted my sisters to help care for

Sophie. She ate all day. True, she clocked a good night's sleep, but I had trouble sometimes distinguishing when one feeding ended and another began. I decided it was time to keep track. I started with the first feeding in the morning and made little slash marks, like the kind prisoners make on a cell-block wall, four down and the fifth one across. When I put Sophie down at night I counted up my scribbles.

The final tally was eighteen.

There it was, eighteen on-demand feedings. I counted, "sixteen, seventeen, *eighteen*." I shouldn't even be revealing this. There are going to be days when your baby is trying to get your supply up and seems to nurse nonstop. I feel like one of those magicians that reveal a big secret on television. Maybe new moms aren't supposed to know this. Would we really nurse?

I called Peter. "Guess how many times I fed your daughter today?"

"Eight, nine?"

"Try eighteen." I stared down at the piece of paper with those sinister slashes. There were so many.

"I don't know what to say."

"If it keeps going like this I'm throwing in the towel. I can't live like this. Something's got to change, because I would rather wean." I had a difficult time understanding why I was bothering with breast-feeding. My misgivings were exacerbated by the fact that I hadn't earned enough stripes to get into the reward period.

"If you feel that way then you need to do what's right for you," Peter said. I was too tired to enter that conversation.

"I'll call you tomorrow." I hung up and fell asleep the moment I hit my feather bed.

Sophie woke me up with her cries. Things had to change. I knew I needed a different approach or I was going to be committed. Taking Jo the police officer's advice, I decided I was going to take it one feeding at a time. There would be no more quick peeks at the cable box's clock. Not a single feeding would be counted. Accepting Sophie's feeding schedule, or lack thereof, was going to be my new goal and the only way I was going to beat the monotony.

Sometime that afternoon I sat down in my glider, wedged my nursing pillow in place, and nursed Sophie. There is a state of being when I'm driving a car and I realize I'm driving, or some part of my brain is driving, but I am not actively thinking about driving. It can be like that with horseback riding or cross-country skiing. It's auto-pilot, but I preferred to look at it in a Far Eastern Zen sort of way. You just do what you're doing without the neurosis.

When Sophie popped off on her own I automatically burped her. I got up from the chair and continued my day. I wrote some e-mails, ordered some baby things from a catalog, and fed Sophie several more times.

I know this isn't possible but my Eureka moment happened gradually.

Somehow in the course of that day, two months into motherhood, nursing had gotten easy. I had fed Sophie several times without the slightest of thought. By not counting feedings, by not looking at the clock, they didn't carry the same weight. No mantra played in my head, I didn't remind myself, "nipple to nose." My wrist kept straight. I didn't think about how to bring her in, I didn't feel a pinch or discomfort. Beyond my cautious relief was my epiphany. I had just entered the Reward Period.

I HAD this "I must tell the others" urgency to my afternoon walk. Peter wouldn't be home for another day but I felt confident enough to put Sophie in the carrier and bring our dog out as well. On my own I could approach new moms at will. There are so many false guarantees in life, like the posters and stickers I see in my neighborhood that promise $50,000 a year from working at home or the ads about instant weight loss.

Now I was a true believer: Yes, yes, they told me nursing would get easier and it did. I'm living proof.

The slow progression to easy had been anticlimactic, but sometimes that's the way easy happens. Out on my walk I didn't run into a single soul, not any of my new mommy friends, not any new moms. It was just that time on a summer afternoon when no one is out on the streets. I called Peter and got his cell phone's voice mail, "Hi there, nursing just got a whole lot easier. This is your wife in case you haven't guessed. Just wanted to let you know things are going much better. Can't wait till you come home." I left several messages on the machines of friends and family. "Hey there, it's Lisa, just wanted to let you know things are going really well, with nursing and everything."

Next I hit the e-mail. "How are things with you? Nursing is going well, much better," I'd write. Who cared how nursing was going for me? My single friends never inquired, but I kept them posted as well. I couldn't wait to see the mommy group, or more truthfully tell the mommy group. It was easy, hallelujah.

I was happy to see the next day's feedings were easy, too. I learned how to lean back, relax, and the calm of victory came over me. Look at me, I'm nursing. With nursing being so difficult I had lived the last two months in the moment. Time passed, the days slipped by, I flipped the months of my calendar, but I was living in an unending here and now. Time was going to pass again without counting feedings or pain levels. I was free of that.

I spent most of the morning with my sisters. Both of them liked to do impressions of me nursing. It was a shtick that always made me laugh.

"Oh, I'm so engorged," Anne kept saying.

"No, I'm engorged," Edith would retort.

"No, I'm engorged," Anne would shoot back. They saw no need to move on to new material.

"Look at me delatch," Edith would say, holding a pretend baby. She would then stick her finger down in her mouth and pull it out slowly. It was a sick version of the way I wet my finger to delatch Sophie. It was funny, but sick.

PETER'S FLIGHT was scheduled to land the following evening. I planned to celebrate a belated Father's Day, his first. I spent a whole afternoon baking a carrot cake, his favorite. Do not attempt this. I would grate the carrots, nurse Sophie, measure out the dry ingredients, nurse Sophie, and so on. It made for frustrating baking. I would get my rhythm, and then I would hear the beginnings of her hunger sounds. They would get louder and louder, until I couldn't take it anymore, even though I just had to drop in a teaspoon of vanilla and pour the batter into the pans. No, with the oven at the right temperature all would have to be on hold until I finished the feeding.

Peter loved the cake, however, without being there to witness the Herculean effort that was needed to make it there was no way he could have fully appreciated its existence. Peter's absence was felt in many ways. I missed him and was beyond happy to see him come through our front door. It wasn't just that I needed his help to walk the dog or change a diaper. I missed him. And though he had only been gone four days he kept saying how much bigger Sophie had grown. She recognized him at once and tried to tell him something in her crib talk.

WE WENT OUT for our evening walk. It was still early enough and, yes, we brought our dog.

146

Once out on the streets any new mom within a two-block radius was fair game. Ignoring pleas from Peter I spotted one.

"Twelve o'clock," I told him.

"Please don't." He had witnessed the complete transformation. And though I would not count myself among women who claim to love nursing, I found it difficult to fathom how easy nursing had actually gotten. My instinct was to spread the word.

"Hi there. Are you nursing?"

"Yes." The woman looked a bit trim for a new mom, her jet-black hair looked done. Was that a blow out? I took note of hair color and her complexion. A friend of mine was convinced the blond and fair had more sensitive skin and therefore were at a disadvantage when it came to nursing. I wasn't sure if her theory was at all true, but I had been taking a mental survey of mothers for the last month.

"How's it going?"

"Really well, she latched on great."

"Wow, you know I had so many problems."

"Really? She's five weeks, and doing wonderfully," she bragged. "It was like kismet in the hospital, never had a problem." I still felt obliged to fill her in on the mother's group, after all I had asked her if she was nursing.

"Good luck, you look wonderful."

"Thanks. Good luck to you too. I'm Barbara."

"I'm Lisa. Hope to see you around," I called to her back as she whisked off.

"Sure it's going well," I said under my breath in my most cynical tone.

"Maybe it is." Peter seemed to buy her story.

"Perhaps." Again I used the voice of doubt. My good talents were wasted on those new moms who didn't need my help. I was looking for the kind of new mom who might pull out a pen from her diaper bag to jot down notes. That was my kind of new mom.

WHEN WE returned home from our walk, Peter unpacked his bag. "What happened on *General Hospital?*" he asked me. He must have used that line half a dozen times since I had Sophie.

"Your material's getting old," I told him. He liked to portray my maternity leave as an excuse to watch daytime television, which I never did. "What do you think I do all day? Do you have any idea of all the stuff I had to do while you were off on your little vacation?" I, in turn, portrayed his work as a vacation. He and his life had stayed the same where my life had changed completely. "I walked the dog, did the laundry, fed your daughter, changed every diaper. If you were a woman, I bet you couldn't hack breast-feeding."

"Ouch, I'm so insulted." He mocked hurt. I don't think he'd really heard what I said. "Please, you have it easy being home." That's when his Father's Day carrot cake ended up in the trash.

We had a truce before we went to bed with him saying sorry. I came to realize that he would never fully appreciate or grasp what being a new nursing mom was like and somehow for the sake of our marriage I needed to accept that. He stopped making those jokes and I haven't made a carrot cake since.

It would be two more days until the mother's group got together again. I couldn't wait. Nursing had gotten easier.

Chapter 12

The Other Thing
Behind a Nursing Mom . . .

TWENTY-SIX POUNDS. That was how much weight I had lost since Sophie was born. I lost all twenty-six pounds during the first two weeks of her life and I had eighteen more to go. Sophie was on her way to being three months old, and nothing had budged. Because I nursed I had the benefit of a uterus that contracted down to its former size. It did that faster than it would have if I had bottle-fed. But who sees my uterus? A real incentive for ladies to nurse would be a quickly contracting behind. As for the claim of getting one's figure back sooner through breast-feeding? That was not my experience.

Not everything gets sucked out through nursing. Brownies, ice cream, and candy seemed to stay. Things went in and found a spot on my stomach, and most notably my rear end. I had ordered several warm-up suits. The first step toward actually exercising is buying the right clothes. I ordered everything in large. The loose pants that were supposed to have a relaxed fit bulged at every seam. The vision I had of myself wasn't at all what I saw in the mirror. Worse was the side view. Was that really me? There it was, a thing that created a shelflike apparatus that hung off my back. How did it get like that?

I had been afflicted with New Mom's Ass.

A college-educated woman I'd met told me that nursing mothers store milk in their butts. She said it with a straight face. I couldn't wait to fact check with Ilana on that point. "No, one doesn't store breast milk there, but breast-feeding women do store fat differently. Some do see it on their backside." I know I did. It was a small miracle that I was able to pull up a pair of size fourteen stretchy pants.

I felt ugly, but I couldn't stay in the apartment until I looked better. Besides I had a dentist appointment. I had avoided getting a filling my entire pregnancy and I couldn't put it off any longer. Though we lived in Brooklyn, because we're crazy we went to a dentist in Ardsley, New York, two bridges and an hour's drive away. Actually, when our dentist moved his practice to Ardsley we went with him. It's a cute suburban town on the border with Yonkers. We brought our dog along, not because we love the way she sheds in the car, but because we had planned to visit my folks after my appointment. Since we couldn't bring the dog inside the dentist's, Peter took a seat on the bench just outside of the office to sit with Halley. First I had my tooth filled and then while Peter's teeth were being cleaned I took my turn outside on the bench. I tied Halley's leash onto one of the bench's slats, put the pillow around my waist, and brought Sophie in to nurse. I don't remember feeling terribly self-conscious. Perhaps because I didn't think anyone would notice me there on a bench off a side street.

I hadn't been sitting there for more than a few minutes when two men walked by. One called over to me, "Yumm . . . I had some of that last night!" They were standing only a few feet away, but felt safe enough to heckle. I was dumbfounded. They weren't kids and they weren't teenagers. They were everyday suburban men. They laughed and walked on. About two minutes later two other men walked by.

"I'd like some of that," one of them said and walked on. Who knew the only two lewd comments I experienced the entire time I nursed Sophie would be within five minutes of each other? Sure I was feeling like a fatty, but I knew nothing was going to intimidate me. I also received a lot of positive comments when I nursed Sophie.

"She's getting fed very well. Good for you," a middle-aged woman said to me when she saw me nursing at a restaurant.

"That's a well-nourished baby," another lady told me. Women said wonderful things to breast-feeding mothers. And the one I received most was, "Good for you." Two creepy comments didn't stack up against that. Still, the experience gave me pause before I would nurse again in unknown territory.

SO WHEN Peter came home one night with the big news that a book editor friend of his had invited the whole family over for dinner, my only hesitation was the idea of having to nurse in close quarters in front of strangers. "But they're French," Peter assured me.

"Right." I was more than happy to agree with Peter, though neither of us knew anything about the French and nursing. Our honeymoon had been in Paris, but we were a self-absorbed couple paying little attention to mothers and children, much less a nursing mother. But we both assumed Europeans must be more enlightened when it came to breast-feeding.

It was one of those humid hotter-than-hell nights. Stepping out of our air-conditioned Camry, I had a single thought on my mind. "I hope they have air-conditioning."

"They're on the top floor," Peter said as he looked down on a scrap piece of paper. I looked up to the top-floor windows. As far as I could tell, there wasn't an air conditioner in sight. Before I could say anything, Peter rang the bell.

"Doesn't look like they have air-conditioning."

"Maybe they're in the back." The glass was always half full with Peter.

I hated my outfit. I couldn't shake my mom look. Lacking any sense of style, I wore the only non-drawstring pants that fit. As for the shirt, my chest was still several cup sizes bigger than my former self, so button-downs were out of the question. I wore a T-shirt that was a bit too tight to pull off. When I left the house I thought it was slimming, but when I sat down my new mommy roll was revealed. So much for fashion.

However hot it was outside, add about ten degrees and that's how hot it was inside. This could have been because the apartment was on the top floor or because they had their oven and several burners going. They were cooking some kind of stew.

The couple had another guest, a twenty-something man. They were all smoking. I had nursed Sophie just before we left in an attempt to stave off nursing as much as I could. Beware of hot days and nursing. Your baby sweats, you sweat. Your baby's thirsty, you're thirsty. Your baby drinks, you drink more. Sophie was ready to nurse almost as soon as we arrived.

"You're feeling hot? I have a fan," said the hostess.

"That would be great," I said, wiping my forehead with a tissue.

Sitting away from the cigarette smoke and closest to the window, I was clearly not the most social guest. I was the ghost of parenthood future. I noticed people often stopped conversing with me once I latched Sophie on to my breast. What else could they say? And I feeling hot and ugly was too preoccupied with my sweating to say, "How 'bout those Yanks." There was a giant disconnect. I was having an out-of-body experience. I missed my new mommy friends. In an effort to seem less freakish, I left the pillow at home, which of course made nursing all the more of a hunched affair. Fresh from the lewd comments I received outside my dentist's office I wasn't feeling that great, not about nursing, not about being in that moronic inferno of a dinner party. The awkwardness that came from nursing in front of others, especially strangers who were childless was inescapable for

152

me—even if they were French. They weren't rude. The hostess tried to make small talk, but they just didn't know what to do with me. She worked a little in television so we played the game where you try and find somebody you know in common.

Under different circumstances, the evening would have been fun. Sitting by myself, I felt so unhappy with my new persona. It wasn't a feeling that made me want to wean Sophie, but I wanted to feel good again, about myself, my new self, my mommy self. I made a resolution in that apartment that night: "I've got to lose this weight."

IF A PAMPHLET had anything to do with new mothers, I grabbed it. There were fliers for new-mother support groups, and several for mommy-and-me yoga classes. Feeling adventurous, I set my sights on the yoga. I still was unable to accept how much longer getting everywhere with the baby took. With the baby, the diaper bag, and my new Maclaren stroller, which I had discovered could go quite fast without worry of bouncing the baby out, I was chronically late to everything. Somehow, even with the extra fifteen minutes I allowed myself, I was late. I was sweating up a storm just filling out the sign-in sheet. I removed my shoes. Since my new sweatpants still didn't fit I was once again in my polo and khakis.

Pulling back the velvet curtain I immediately wanted to make a U-turn, but they had all seen my theatrical entrance. Too late to turn around, I scolded myself for not peeking first. It wasn't the class I thought it was. I was used to the walking-wounded gals of my breast-feeding support group. The ladies in the class were thin, very thin and in impossible poses.

"Sorry I'm late," I mouthed to the instructor.

"C-section?" the instructor mouthed back at me. I hated the class right away and I hated the instructor even more. Where was all the good yoga love?

"No, I'm just out of shape." I wanted to give her a proviso, *this* wasn't my body, I was just borrowing it for the postpartum period. Weren't we all out of shape after having a baby? Taking a good look at the model-type moms in the class, I asked the instructor, "Is this the advanced mommy-and-me yoga? These women look like they're in incredible shape."

"Did you hear that, class? She just said you were all in incredible shape." Turning toward me she let me in on a little secret. "Most of them took my prenatal class." There wasn't anything more to say.

What was that C-section comment supposed to mean? Wasn't I allowed to be out of shape after a vaginal birth? Wasn't I entitled to be a little winded and flabby? Unrolling my mat out on the floor I was seething. I placed Sophie on the blanket in front of me. The woman next to me was rail thin, fully extended in some pose. Her son looked to be the same age as Sophie. Turning my anger into disgust with my own body I tried to bend forward. The splint on my wrist was visible, though the instructor didn't seem to notice *that*. Perhaps she was blindsided by my ass. Was bending forward safe? I didn't anticipate how much wrist action was required to do yoga. I didn't want to just give up, though it was obvious I already missed the easy stuff. I should have just walked out.

The stress of being in that class with all of my hormones out of whack made me perspire profusely.

"Are you ready to try, Dahlia?" the instructor asked a well-tanned mother with a tiny newborn.

"I think so. She's only three weeks, but I'm dying to try, it's been forever." That's right, she was out of the house with a three-week-old. Dahlia got up from her mat, walked over to the wall, threw down some pillow, and did a handstand inversion. There was no New Mom's Ass on her.

My simple desire to stretch a few muscles had somehow subjected me to the cool, thin mom dog-and-pony show. I bet those women weren't nursing their babies. As class wrapped up, I overheard their conversations.

"With my last baby the nursing bras were so ugly. I found this store, Boing Boing in Park Slope, and they have the greatest selection of nursing bras, some really sexy ones." She pulled back her tee and revealed a lacy black thing. It was then that I understood. Cool moms hung out at advanced baby yoga, while I was busy bonding at the breast-feeding support group. The cool moms were looking for the sexy nursing bras (isn't that an oxymoron?) while I wore cabbage.

The whole excursion had made me hungry. By the time I made it back down to the street I was starving. With my last drop of energy I pushed Sophie's stroller to my favorite specialty food store, Lassen and Hennings. I quickly purchased a sandwich, soda, and large cookie. There I was on the corner of Henry and Montague. I couldn't wait till I was home or found a bench, no, I stood over Sophie's stroller taking large unladylike bites out of my Waldorf Chicken Sandwich. With my mouth full I could barely say hello when that Dahlia strutted by. Her baby was tucked in her sling and in both hands were bags of groceries. She smiled at me and for that I hated her.

THE NEXT DAY was the breast-feeding support group. Walking into the meeting made me exhale in that way you do when you walk through your front door. True, the meetings were no longer as urgent as they used to be, as most of us had entered our Reward Period. There was always a new mom who we would all cheer on with our words of support or personal story. The new mom at this meeting was a trim young woman without a baby. She didn't look pregnant nor did she look like she had recently given birth.

155

I overheard her telling Rachel that her son was in the neonatal ward. He was born ten weeks early, but she was pumping and intended to nurse her son.

"You know I was just beginning to show, so when my water broke and I had to have a C-section, I just wasn't that big."

"Wait, when did you have a baby?" I had to know, she looked like a normal person. Not a new mom who had just gone through the most traumatic of experiences.

"Last week," she told everyone.

"Congratulations, that's really amazing you are going to pump," Rachel said.

"I've just started and it's going well."

"Get the Classic," I instructed in my do-what-I-say-or-else voice. We were all inspired by any new mom who found her way to the group. I used to think it was the more experienced moms who were inspiring, see they made it through, they got educated, they sought out help and got it. Now, I was repeatedly in awe of any new mom who came into our circle of chairs in the windowless room off of the maternity ward. You found it. Wow, don't give up. There was one mom who was supplementing and pumping, she recently had surgery and *still* nursed her child.

When I first began going it was sometimes difficult to get a word in or ask a question. Now, since most of us were old pros at nursing there sometimes was a lull in conversation, that's when another type of question was asked, the "stump the lactation consultant" kind.

"If I lived solely on my own breast milk, how long would I last?" I asked. I had watched too much *Survivor*. Ilana took this question very seriously.

"Well, breast milk is very nutritious, so you would be able to go a while," Ilana said. Good to know.

I also felt obliged to report on my own unscientific findings regarding the connection between a Starbuck's Frappachino and a baby's crankiness. I believed there was a connection. And there was always someone at the group who would ask, "Has anyone tasted it yet?" Nearly everyone I knew had. "It's a bit like almondine," a friend once told me. I had yet to gulp any. As hungry and thirsty as I was, breast milk didn't appeal to me.

We left en masse from the hospital. We made sure the mothers' group met twice a week all through the summer. We took in matinees, went on field trips, tried new restaurants, and occasionally indulged at Ben and Jerry's, all with our babies in tow. It felt like camp, but for breast-feeders, and it was not uncommon for one of our afternoons to last four or five hours. I know I have such fond memories of Sophie's first year because of those afternoons. What I didn't fully appreciate at the time was how privileged I was to be part of a nursing mom's group. We were inclusive and would not have turned away a woman who chose to bottle-feed. It's just that our group formed organically out of the support group. And it was that shared experience of nursing that bonded us together.

I proposed that our next field trip was going to be to the sexy nursing-bra store, Boing Boing. It was also my chance to dish and give all the gory details about the mommy-and-me yoga class.

"If you're all around next week, we should all go together."

"Sounds advanced." Jamie was hesitant. I had made a huge mistake in telling them about the mom who did a headstand inversion three weeks after giving birth. But in my own warped thinking, I believed that if I got my mothers' group to attend next Tuesday's mommy-and-me yoga, the class wouldn't be as difficult. Somehow they all agreed to go.

We walked in. The heat immediately got us. It was easily more than a hundred degrees in the studio. I put my hair up in a ponytail and noticed I was holding a fistful of strands of my own hair. The slightest yank seemed to pull out dozens. There was no mistaking it. I was losing my hair. Those wacky hormones.

The instructor turned on the air-conditioning and promised that the room would cool down in minutes. There were only two moms from last week's class, a good thing. Obviously the instructor would tailor the class to our level.

"If it doesn't cool down soon I'm not going to stay." Norma held Lilly and waited while standing. I recognized someone else, Barbara, the "no problems nursing mom." There she was with her tiny bundle.

"I love her class," Barbara confided to me. That was strike two. I set my mat down next to Barbara to be polite.

Right away the instructor went into her routine. She showed no mercy. I had thought the class was difficult because I had missed the warm-up. Not so. The class started at an advanced level right away. She was going to shake us down to find out who was a tourist.

With all the warmth of a corrections officer the instructor started in on my mommy group. "This is a sorry group of mothers. Come on people, you have to bring those strollers up those subway stairs." My mothers had been ensnared in a trap of sorts. Maybe I needed the affirmation that I wasn't the only sorry mother, that I had company in my out-of-shape postpartum state and I wasn't alone. It was the cool skinny moms that were a minority. It was obvious those moms *had* issues. I glanced over at Barbara. She was bending and twisting the class away. There was no chance I was going to like this lady. When I glanced over at Jamie, she mouthed the word "help." Norma rolled her eyes. There was one acceptable way out of doing mommy-and-me yoga—nursing. I picked up Sophie and sat down against the wall. She wasn't hungry, but with a little encouragement, "Eat or I'll have to finish this god-forsaken class," I latched her on. Sophie nursed. What an adorable gorgeous baby. I looked down at her and forgot that I was using her to get out of yoga, that I was in an overheated class with an overheated instructor.

"Come on mommies, New York City is a tough place, you need to stay in shape." Soon Jamie and Norma were nursing as well.

When the class was finished, I rejoined for the quite meditation at the end when everyone laid down on their mats. Barbara turned to me. "Wasn't that awesome?"

"Yeah," I agreed.

Once we were out on the street and I was with the inner circle of my mommy group we all concurred about the rotten treatment we'd received.

"I didn't need to spend fifteen bucks to be told I'm in sorry shape."

"She was awful," Jamie said.

"Did you hear how she insulted us? I mean I took prenatal yoga in the city and that instructor let everyone go at her own speed." Norma was miffed.

"We were a sorry group of mothers? Who is that woman?" Secretly relieved that I wasn't alone in my surprise at the class's difficulty I also felt some guilt about subjecting my new mommy friends to that barrage of ill will. We continued to dish on our creepy instructor. We talked about joining gyms and exercise.

"Maybe we should all do a stroller walk," Norma suggested. It was a good idea.

"We should set up a time, like on Saturday mornings," Jamie added. At least now we had a plan. What a relief. We would all lose weight together. We headed on to our favorite deli and then on to Ben and Jerry's for a light snack.

MONTHS LATER at my very first gentle yoga class, I waited patiently as everyone recounted their tale of woe and what brought them to the class. I tried to decide just how to phrase, "I couldn't hack mommy-and-me yoga." One woman went on and on in graphic detail about a car accident. The next man had a workplace injury and there was another woman who went into the effects of old age on every nook and cranny of her body. There were sad tales of injuries and falls. Perhaps a better name for the class would have been geriatric yoga.

It was my turn. I just came out with it. "I couldn't really keep up in the mommy-and-me yoga class."

"Awe . . ." that was the chorus of my gentle yoga classmates. The woman hit by a car didn't get an "awe." That was how pathetic my story was.

"Well, tell me what is that splint on your wrist? Are you suffering from carpal tunnel?" the gentle yoga instructor wanted to know.

"Yes, it started in pregnancy, but was aggravated by nursing."

"Awe . . ." the class continued their pity party.

"You aren't going to be able to do most of what we do here in this class, but I'll show you some alternate poses." Finally there was an instructor with a heart.

"Oh, I didn't realize."

I took one more class before giving up yoga altogether.

Chapter 13

The Purgatory of Part-time Work

BY THE END of the summer Sophie was four months old and most of the moms from the mothers' group were preparing to return to work full-time. Before Sophie was born I had looked down on those women who chose to stay home with their children. I know that's unfair, but I felt that "stay-at-home mom" was a euphemism for "housewife," and there was nothing lower than a housewife. My mother had worked outside the home when I was growing up. Her mother had worked as well. Maybe it was growing up in the seventies and eighties. My early years were on the tail end of the women's movement and in the eighties there were media images everywhere of women in suits holding briefcases in one hand and a baby or frying pan in the other. The myth of "having it all" was drilled into my head. True my mother was exhausted. It was a lot having three kids and working full-time. But that was all I knew. And I certainly couldn't see myself staying home.

My hope in starting my company was to have the freedom to be a mom and have a flexible schedule. I boasted how "I knew myself," and I was one of those people who loved to work. I loved coming home by car service at eleven o'clock at night, and I wasn't used to weekends without work. The pregnancy had slowed down my pace. I was careful not to work the long hours, but I figured that I would be back at full force as soon as I recovered from delivery.

Since I was a partner in my production company I didn't take a complete maternity leave, which at times was difficult. I even signed a few checks in my recovery room at the hospital, which was nuts. But that was my life as a small-business owner. There were taxes to pay and calls to return. I spent most of Sophie's naps dealing with work-related business. I took meetings here and there. I wasn't ready to hire a sitter full-time, but I needed help with Sophie two to three times a week. My mom's antique business was picking up and she had less time to lend me by early August. I made a deal with my younger sister, Edith. She was on break from college, where she was earning an MFA, and she was still without a job. With my flexible hours and Edith's studio schedule we saw the situation as temporary, but mutually beneficial. Edith would watch Sophie for ten dollars an hour. Striking a business deal with family is not something I usually contemplated but I did see how much Sophie liked her aunt. In September Edith would be going back to school and then I would find a full-time sitter.

And just as I had never really been on leave, I also didn't go back full-time right away. I began going into my Midtown office when Sophie was little more than six weeks old. I was doing a day or two a week. I still had the occasional shoot to do and I was waiting to hear if the series was going to be renewed. Ambivalent wasn't the right word for how I felt about working. I was conflicted. Conflicted about getting full-time child care, conflicted over leaving Sophie, conflicted about staying in television. But I could usually suppress those feelings while I was with my mommy friends. Nursing away, blabbing about our husbands, our in-laws, our bodies, and our babies. The park was my refuge.

When my cell phone would ring I would be yanked out of my afternoon Xanadu. After making a few recommendations to the producer I would rejoin the others, hoping not to be interrupted again. Since summer would soon be over, most of our conversations were about work. Two of the moms said they were ready to return. One woman I knew through a friend said she loved going back to work so she could be "a real person again."

A year earlier I had been on the fence about continuing the work I was doing. I wanted a change, but things with the company were going well. I had a wait-and-see attitude. With the baby, those feelings of wanting to leave television production returned. I personally knew few women who worked in production and had children. The one woman I did know with children in the business told me she liked working so she could rest, being at home was exhausting.

AT THE breast-feeding support group the conversation focused on how to pump at work. "I read that nursing is a civil right in New York State. And that your employer needs to make a private place available for pumping." I had just read *Breast-feeding and the Working Mother* by Diane Mason and Diane Ingersoll.

"I think that's true. As far as nursing goes, you can nurse anywhere in New York and no one can tell you to stop." Norma read up on the laws as well.

"But it isn't a civil right everywhere?" Jamie asked.

"I don't believe so but in New York it is," Norma said.

"I think you need to check state to state," Ilana said.

"Are you supposed to look at a photo of your baby when you pump? I noticed my new Pump In Style had a little frame on the flap for a picture." Peter recently returned my Classic, which was way too heavy to carry, much less take on a subway to work. For a little under three hundred dollars I purchased the Medela Pump In Style Traveler.

"Some women say looking at a photo helps them when they pump. You should try it, see if it helps," Ilana suggested.

Feeling in the mood to share, I wanted to tell the rest of the group about the four-month milestone. It was standing-room-only at the meeting, and we had asked so many questions we hadn't even begun the introductions. I had never seen so many moms at the breast-feeding support group.

After several people introduced themselves, it was my turn. "I'm Lisa and this is Sophie. Sophie is four months. When she was born and I was having trouble nursing her, four months was my goal. And now here we are." Just like that I heard a crack in the back of my throat. Was I going to break down in tears at the group? Over the summer there had been several moms who had the waterworks going, but not me. I had wanted to say something like here we are and I plan to go another eight months to make a year. But I didn't dare say any more. I hoped no one noticed that crack in my voice. I sat there quietly and tried to smile. That was a close one.

It was my badge of honor that I had kept things light, funny, and away from the gestalt of my new-mom experience. I was still in it, still finding my way, and if I let the vulnerability take over I wasn't sure how far I would go.

We left the meeting and no one said anything. So Norma once again gave us the details of her tear.

I wasn't sure if becoming a mother had made me weak, or was really breaking the tough façade I had constructed years ago.

MY SOLUTION for new motherhood and to keep my job was to work part-time. My logic followed this trajectory: if the series was picked up for another season I would be ready, and if the series wasn't renewed, then I was laying the foundation developing new shows. With my wrists shot I knew I wasn't going to be doing any more camera work. I was going to do nine-to-five three days a week, and depending on what work came in the fall I would increase the schedule. Calls for work were still coming in, and I almost had to turn down a job because I feared not being ready to take it on.

THERE WAS one guy who shared office space on the same floor as my office. His wife recently had a baby. He was heavyset but his bigness made him seem like a Teddy bear. He came into my office on one of my first days back.

"Mazel Tov, I'm so excited for you," I told him.

He turned to me and with a straight face said, "I'd better get laid soon or I don't know what I'm going to do. I need sex." Was that new-daddy talk? While us gals were off trying to nurse our babies, the guys were wondering where to get laid?

The jokes at the office never seemed lewd before, but now I wanted to say, "Hey, take you and your potty mouth and get out of my office, I'm someone's mommy."

Instead I smiled at the guy and said, "I'm really busy with work and this isn't appropriate." He no longer seemed like a Teddy bear.

New moms do at some point talk about sex, but it's usually after the six-week postpartum period. There was one mom who came to the group infrequently who offered up that she and her husband started having sex five weeks after she delivered her baby boy.

"I couldn't do that," I told her. I wasn't a prude, I hadn't become asexual, I just wasn't ready at five weeks.

"Oh please, my husband would leave me," she said. I kept waiting for her to laugh and say she was kidding but she didn't. One mom announced with pride that her "shop" had opened again. And there were several other moms who felt obliged to report when things were back in business. For me, all good things happened when I entered that reward period. Once nursing was easy, I wasn't as tense about everything else, though it was going to take time to get back to where Peter and I once were. The most difficult thing was how I felt about myself. I had yet to feel pretty again, much less sexy.

BY NOT being in the office every day I was constantly missing calls. I would call back, they wouldn't be in, they would call me back and I was out with the baby. Not a single business suit fit. I came into the office in khakis and polo shirts and prayed I wouldn't run into anyone I knew. Without heels and a great outfit, dressing for work wasn't what it used to be. If I told someone I had child care on Mondays, Wednesdays, and Fridays they would schedule a meeting on Tuesday or Thursday. The line between home and work blurred into this inefficient pattern of missed calls and rescheduled meetings. That was the purgatory of part-time work.

My younger sister, Edith, often met me at my office. I would hand over Sophie and then head out for a meeting. It usually went well, unless Sophie freaked out and disrupted the office, which did happen.

Since I was mainly doing development much of my business was speculative. When we had a lot of work I never noticed how much time was spent developing a project. Since things had slowed down, every moment at work cost me money, ten dollars an hour to be exact. I was paying ten dollars an hour for every meeting, every business lunch, the whole day added up. Yes, I still received a salary but everything had a different perspective. It wasn't just the cost of child care. There was something else going on. Things that once seemed important and pressing were downgraded to drudgery or annoyance.

"How many ounces did she take in today?" I'd ask Edith if she was watching Sophie back in Brooklyn. She would give me a number, two, three, etc . . . Then I would close the door to my cubbylike office and pump the same amount. The best part of my Pump In Style Traveler was its backpack carrying case. It was comfortable and it didn't look like a breast pump. On one of my first days back at work I took the elevator with a twenty-something woman.

"I love your backpack," she told me.

"You know what it is?" I couldn't help myself. It had been so long since someone gave me a compliment that I was thrilled even if it was for my breast pump, which now was the most stylish thing about me.

"No, what is it?" She looked perplexed and I could tell she regretted giving me the compliment.

"It's a breast pump."

"Oh, I'm so embarrassed." She laughed.

"You made my day." The doors opened and I walked out. Immediately I went around the office and told everyone in sight that a woman in the elevator complimented my breast pump.

MY HOPE had been to go into more production, though each day I grew more apprehensive to commit to anything long-term. I chalked up my feelings as the baby blues. My mommy friends e-mailed about their transition back to work. Norma wrote about seeing a mom push a stroller down the street while on her lunch break. It had been Norma's first day back at work and that image brought her to tears. On the other hand, Rachel had taken a seven-month maternity leave and loved being back at work. She loved her office and was happy to see all her music downloads were still in her hard drive. I kept waiting for my I-love-being-back-at-work feeling to kick in.

Toward the end of August we all met up one last time at the breast-feeding support group. I bought a throwaway camera at the hospital's gift shop. I wanted a group photo for Sophie's baby book.

Perhaps women were meant to sit in circles, sharing their experiences. I once asked Ilana what I would have done if I lived in a village hundreds of years ago without a breast pump. As she explained, the other mothers would have helped. Had I been engorged the other mothers would have nursed my child. I in turn would have nursed an older child to drain my breast. In this day and age of latex gloves and the biohazard that has become our fluids it is incomprehensible, but theoretically I understood. Maybe that is why sitting with those women learning to nurse had felt right, the way a campfire does, something primal and warm.

I knew there would be more field trips and our Saturday stroller walks but saying good-bye that last meeting was difficult. Together with our babies we posed for a photo.

MOVING FORWARD with work I scheduled a meeting with an agent. A colleague of mine told me the agent was interested in representing the company so I figured I had nothing to lose. I drove in and parked at some super-expensive parking lot. Edith met me at my office. I gave her Sophie, a bottle, and the stroller. Then the phone rang. The meeting had been canceled. Without the baby, a canceled meeting wouldn't have made a dent in my day, but it nearly brought me to tears. Going all the way into the city with the baby was work. I should have left her home with Edith, but thought bringing her in would be easier. I was getting breast pump fatigue and was trying to avoid pumping when possible. The meeting was rescheduled and a week later I came into the office again. And once again I set Edith up with the bottle and stroller.

The agent's office was located on the high floor of a Midtown building. The main offices were über-modern, but the agent's office was dusty. On the wall hung a poster of an independent film from the early nineties. His beard was gray, the same color as his skin. The only shiny thing in his office was his head.

"Great seeing you again."

"You had a kid right?"

"She's almost five months old."

"I didn't ask you how old she was, I asked if you had a kid."

I wanted to leave the office right there and then, but a friend had set up the meeting, so an early exit wasn't an option.

"So you wanted to meet about the company?"

"I did? That's news to me," he said.

The meeting pretty much went like that. I had no idea why I was there except to be on the receiving end of his bitter rhetoric. And I don't know why I continued to be polite. I didn't like how I looked in my loose white linen shirt. Feeling vulnerable, I wasn't myself.

The giant thought in my mind, perhaps it is the thought that passes through every working mom's consciousness was, "Why am I paying someone ten dollars an hour to watch my baby while I'm sitting here with this asshole?" It was a crystalline moment.

When the meeting ended I felt my milk let-down.

"Great seeing you," he called to me as I made my way out of the office.

Edith reported that Sophie didn't want the bottle. She cried or wailed for nearly fifteen minutes. A fact that everyone in the office noted.

"Why didn't you take her outside? Don't you know what a nuisance it is to hear a baby cry when you're trying to work?" I was angry

169

more about the meeting than about Sophie's crying. Edith was defensive and couldn't wait to head out.

I went into the lounge, the only private room in the space. I locked the door, sat down, brought Sophie onto my breast, and burst into tears.

BEFORE I LEFT the office I made sure everything was in order. I had been working part-time since Sophie was born and decided it was time for a little vacation. The last two weeks in August were slow anyway. I resolved to return in September. Then I would hire a baby-sitter and work full-time. In the meantime I would enjoy Sophie and not worry about work.

I'd imagined hanging out with my mom friends, but most of the mother's group had gone back to work full-time. In addition, Brooklyn was dead in late August, so the ghost town feel was even greater as I strolled around searching for the summer's familiar faces.

On Wednesday I decided to stop by the breast-feeding support group.

Just as I had done all spring and summer, I made my way through the labyrinth that was the hospital, taking two different elevators to bring me to the maternity ward. I pressed the bell, was buzzed in, and waited for a nurse to lead me into the classroom. Unlike before there wasn't a recognizable face.

"Are you here for the breast-feeding support group?" a short woman with almost purple hair asked.

"Yes. Is Ilana here?"

"I'm Jenny, I'm the new leader."

It was too late to back out. I had no idea that Ilana and Laura gave the reins of the breast-feeding support group to someone else. I was struck by how unfamiliar the room was without my friends. It

170

shouldn't have been a surprise since they had all gone back to work, but I had hoped I'd know someone. All the new faces and newborn babies brought the realization that my special summer was officially over. Someone was sitting in my usual chair so I took my place next to Jenny.

"Why don't we go around the room and introduce ourselves?" Jenny motioned to one of the other moms.

"I'm Ethel and this is Conner," a mousy mom with frizzy hair said. She was the one sitting in my usual seat. "He's three weeks old."

"I'm Joanna and this is Emma," said a blond woman who appeared to be in great shape. "She's almost two months old." Two months, where has she been keeping herself? She finally made it to the group, how quaint. I should have been supportive, saying something like, "It's amazing you're here," but I didn't. Another mom made her introduction, but by then it was all white noise to me, I was waiting for my turn. I had felt out of place at the office, and now I felt out of place at the group.

"My name is Lisa and this is Sophie, and . . ." Inhaling slowly, my breath got caught somewhere between my lips and my lungs. My cheeks warmed with blood. "Usually my friends are all here." There it was, a tear tricked down my cheek, then another. I was going down.

My first rule about the breast-feeding support group was: Don't cry at the breast-feeding support group.

"And you miss your friends?" Jenny asked in a soft soothing voice. My lip quivered so I opted to nod in agreement.

"They were here all summer?" Jenny asked. Again I nodded. Jenny handed me a tissue.

"I can't believe I'm crying," I sniffled. The other mothers stared at me.

It would have been one thing to lose it in the early days, when nursing was so difficult, when we were allowed to go *there*. But there

I was, tears and all crying in front of a bunch of freshman. I got out of there as soon as I politely could. Thank goodness the girls weren't there to witness that sorry display. On second thought I wished they had been there. I wasn't ready to be cut loose. And then there was Sophie. When I got home I took her out of her stroller and she giggled in delight. All I could do was smile back.

Chapter 14

The Comfort of Nursing

PETER HAD ASKED me to join him on a business trip to a Utah writers' conference. Though I had wanted to stay behind in New York, Peter was excited about taking Sophie and me. He planned a mini-vacation after the conference: We would head south from Salt Lake City and spend two nights at a resort on the Colorado River, just above Moab.

My parents had called that morning because they needed a Sophie fix and knew we were leaving town. I had almost finished packing when they arrived. I needed to get out of the house so we headed for the promenade in Brooklyn Heights.

We were all especially proud of Sophie's latest achievement, which was putting her foot in her mouth. And if I danced in front of her she would kick and wiggle her arms. We snapped off several photos of my parents holding Sophie in front of the New York City skyline. Likewise my parents took photos of Peter, Sophie, and me. It was a bright sunny day and we ate outside at a café. Sophie was a complete flirt smiling at the patrons at the other tables. The whole excursion took my mind off our flight the next day. I am always pre-occupied the day before I fly. I've had a fear of flying since my early twenties and had taken Valium the last few times I flew. But I was nursing, so no Valium for me.

We drove our car to the airport and parked it in long-term parking, which took longer than we anticipated. Peter ran ahead with Sophie and her stroller. We made it to our gate with only minutes to spare. We made a spectacle out of ourselves only once. As I was digging for my boarding pass I hung both the diaper bag and my purse on the stroller's handles, and the weight made the stroller flip back. Sophie was startled and cried, but she was okay. I felt terrible. I even heard a woman on a cell phone describe the whole thing, "No the stroller flipped with the baby *in* it." Peter and I exchanged a few testy words but we made up by the time we took our seats.

As per the pediatrician's recommendation I nursed Sophie on takeoff and landing. It is important to do this for several reasons, it calms them, and the motion of sucking helps their ears when they pop. To my surprise I was calm, the very act of nursing worked like Valium for me. Sophie was in the BabyBjörn and slept for most of the flight.

I spent the conference strolling around the hotel, working out in the hotel's gym (with Sophie next to me on a blanket) and e-mailing friends from the mothers' group using my laptop. I was too intimidated to take Sophie around town in our rental car. Peter was busy meeting with prospective writers and speaking on a panel. We were able to take in a few sights but I was doing time until we could head to the resort.

When the conference wrapped up, we drove south, stopping once for lunch. Sophie had yet to start solids, so every time we ate, I simply nursed her. The pediatrician had told me that when Sophie no longer slept through the night or nursed nonstop I would know it was time to start solids, but that until then it was fine to keep nursing her exclusively. There was no water or juice, just me. And being the great travel companion that she was, she slept through the night.

Southern Utah was an alien landscape to my eyes. It reminded me of the Wile E. Coyote cartoons. We arrived late in the afternoon and though it was September, the temperature was well above a hundred, something we hadn't considered when we made our plans.

Part of the resort's appeal was its horses and trail rides. I had thought I would be interested in horseback riding, but I signed Peter up first. Before I was pregnant Peter and I went riding every weekend, but I was hesitant to start again. It seemed too risky for me. "What if I fall off and break my arm, how would I nurse?" I asked Peter. He tried to encourage me, and though the resort's quarter horses were docile, I didn't feel like taking a chance. The next morning he went for a ride.

That afternoon, when the temperature began to drop, we snapped Sophie into the BabyBjörn, grabbed an umbrella, and headed up the trail to Arches National Park's most famous attraction, Delicate Arch.

We reached the arch in a little less than an hour and were surprised by the number of people squeezed into the lookout. Everyone was waiting for the grand finale of the setting sun. The arches of the park had been sculpted by the elements over millions of years. Delicate Arch with the La Sal Mountains in the background looked as improbable as it did beautiful. It was worth the hike. I found a spot to sit down and though there wasn't a great deal of personal space, I nursed Sophie. In the arid dry heat I couldn't gauge how much water she was losing. It seemed like she was nursing more than usual but I wasn't sure. I noticed I was getting a few stares from the other hikers. I was trying to be discreet, and I would have been had Peter not taken several snapshots, all with a flash. "We need photos of you nursing in front of landmarks," Peter joked. I guess they would end up in Sophie's baby book. Peter told me that he thought my nursing Sophie up there on the ledge by Delicate Arch was one of the cooler things he'd witnessed. Have breasts, will travel.

We hiked back to the car by flashlight, just in time to bat away the hundreds of bugs that found us in the parking lot.

Aside from the bug attack, it had been a great getaway. I was so glad we came along. "This was a great vacation," I told Peter. I felt rested. I felt rejuvenated. I was ready to get back to work.

THE FOLLOWING DAY we woke early enough to see the sunrise, which was mind-blowing. I was sorry to leave the resort. I had been so eager to return home but after seeing that sunrise, two days in Moab didn't seem long enough. We had planned to leave around nine in the morning to make our afternoon flight out of Salt Lake. I took a shower after Peter and somehow he had packed all of my clothes and put them in the car. I didn't even have underwear.

"Do you think you could maybe not pack the clothes I'm supposed to wear?"

I was grumpy, my usual mood on the days that I fly. It was time to nurse Sophie. I wanted to make it all the way back to Salt Lake without stopping, so I needed to make sure she was full. I was sitting on the sofa nursing, wearing only a towel when Peter returned empty-handed.

"Where are my clothes?"

"We're not flying today."

"What?"

"Two planes hit the World Trade Center and another crashed into the Pentagon. No one's flying today."

"Why are you telling me this?" I yelled at him and his absurd joke.

"I'm serious, I just went to check out and the guy said no one's flying today."

Peter grabbed the remote. The resort had satellite television. We were able to watch New York City's local news. There on the

176

screen was footage of the second plane going into the south tower. Both towers were the way everyone saw them that day, the way they were carved into our memories. My older sister, Anne, worked three blocks from the World Trade Center and I could think of nothing else. The phones of course were useless. For whatever reason, the only person we could reach was my grandmother in Prospect Harbor, Maine.

"Anne's okay, she just landed in Boston," my grandmother reported. She had landed at Logan International Airport in Boston two minutes after the first plane hit. I was so glad I didn't know she was flying that day. Edith was out in the Hamptons. Not one of my parents' daughters was in the city that day.

Peter was out by the car when the first tower collapsed.

I placed Sophie on the floor. She was on her belly looking up at the television. Peter returned with the luggage. It was clear we weren't going anywhere, at least for the next day.

September eleventh was one of the few times I've seen my husband cry. In between our bouts of near hysteria, the day dragged on with us trying to make phone calls to family members. Peter's cousin lived in TriBeCa, the residential neighborhood above the financial center. She walked across the Brooklyn Bridge and found her parents. Our families were very lucky.

We called our landlord to ask if she could shut the windows in our apartment. We used to be able to see the Twin Towers from our kitchen window. I wished we were home.

Peter's next order of business was to extend our stay. We didn't know when the airports would open again. We would be able to keep our room for one more night then we would have to switch to another cabin. That afternoon we drove into Moab.

"What if we end up in Moab for the rest of our lives?" I asked Peter. As implausible as it seems, that was a legitimate question that day. We had no idea what would happen next.

When I saw the towers fall, I thought about the mothers, about their babies who may or may not have been weaned, about the women who brought their pumps to work. Maybe someone was off pumping. I found myself obsessing over the "what if's" of nursing and death. I thought of Sophie and what would happen if I were gone one day never to return. I thought of the frozen milk in my freezer and how many feedings that might last.

I hadn't seen the world through a mother's eyes like I did that day. I couldn't sleep that night. I kept thinking about the people whose lives ended that day, but I thought most about the mothers.

BECAUSE WE WERE New Yorkers, the behavior of the other guests at the resort seemed inappropriate. Guests were going on trail rides and ordering room service. The landscape was foreign to me. People weren't going to hold a vigil like they were doing back home.

The reports of men impersonating pilots and airport shutdowns kept us in limbo for another day. We didn't know what to do with ourselves. I was able to get online and wrote all of the mothers from the group. Did they get home in time to nurse? There were other thoughts, like was everyone okay? Some of the moms worked on Wall Street.

And what if we had been home? We had a new parents' first-aid kit but that was about as prepared as we were, unless you considered nursing part of an emergency plan. I didn't have to boil bottles. I didn't even need water much less sterile water to mix formula. What if there was a run on formula? Nursing was my disaster plan, except of course if something did happen to me.

178

THERE WAS nothing for us to do but wait. We watched the news in a hypnotic trance. Although there was no new information, the newscasts reminded us that this wasn't a nightmare. It had happened.

That evening our plan began to unfold. We went into Moab and bought a road atlas of North America. Advertised on the back of the atlas was a map of the United States, with its interstate highways and the locations of Best Westerns. The car rental company had waived the fees of one-way returns and we already had unlimited mileage.

Our plan was to leave early the next morning. We wanted to make it as far as Lincoln, Nebraska. The map's timeline estimated a ten-hour ride. On Friday we would leave Lincoln and spend the next night in Davenport, Iowa. From Davenport we would head to Chicago, from there we would head to Detroit. In Detroit we would stay with my aunt and uncle. By Sunday we would leave for my parents who lived in Jersey. Monday was Rosh Hashanah. If all went according to plan we would arrive back in Brooklyn on Tuesday.

The next day we got an early start and headed north. What we didn't account for was the time it took to nurse Sophie. She wasn't quite five months old and still needed to be fed every third hour. When we embarked on the first leg of the trip we promised ourselves that I would never nurse Sophie in a moving car. By that evening just outside Denver there I was. I had crawled into the back seat, unsnapped Sophie out of her car seat and nursed her.

"Drive slow," I told Peter. There was terrible traffic so I dialed the toll-free Best Western number to have them move our reservation from Lincoln to Denver. They booked us in a room at the Best Western right outside the Denver airport, which was quiet that night.

Peter's eyes were bloodshot from all the driving. The rain and traffic made it all the more difficult. What were we thinking? How were we ever going to get home? It was going to take us weeks at our pace. But it was too late to turn back and I couldn't fathom flying again.

The next morning we were back on the road.

"Today we are going to stop every time Sophie needs to nurse."

Again by the late afternoon I found myself in the backseat, nursing. I was buckled in but you could not deny the safety issue of nursing a baby in a moving car.

We felt the most welcomed in the truck stops along the way. The waitresses were especially sympathetic. As they poured coffee they would ask where we were from. "New York City," we'd reply, usually in unison.

"I'm so sorry," they would say.

"We're heading home, been driving since Utah," we would tell them. We would buy gas and strike up conversations with people who had rented cars in New York and were making their way home to LA. We ran into a couple who bought a car in Las Vegas because there were no more rentals. They were making their way back home to Boston. On the highway we saw a minivan with California plates. Inside sat a half dozen men in Oxford shirts and suits. The signs in front of drive-ins, churches, and schools spelled out words of unity and support. "God Bless America." Or "Our hearts are with you New York." Those signs dotted the plains.

I called the toll-free Best Western number one more time and moved our reservation from Davenport to Omaha. It was our second night in a Best Western and the room in Omaha was shabby but we were too tired to complain. We called my parents with the latest on our whereabouts. After nursing Sophie I hooked up my laptop to the outlet and went online. There was e-mail from the mothers' group.

All of the mothers and their families were safe. We had all been unbelievably fortunate.

180

WHEN I SAW the Chicago skyline I knew we were halfway home. I booked us at a Four Seasons in Chicago. After two nights and three days on the road, I thought we should try something new. The best thing about the hotel, aside from it being a Four Seasons, was the crib. It was the first decent crib Sophie had slept in for days. It even had bumpers. They provided diapers and baby items as well.

Since the attacks, we had used our downtime to catch up with the news on CNN, so to splash around in the hotel's pool didn't feel right. But Peter's back was stiff from the hours of driving and we all needed to unwind. Sophie wore her little purple gingham bathing suit, Peter stretched out, and I dipped Sophie in the water. She loved the pool, which we had all to ourselves. Sophie was oblivious to all that had happened. "Who's our little swimmer?" I asked her. She kicked her feet and splashed the water with her hands. She took such pleasure in it. Peter and I handed her back and forth moving her through the water. We all felt better.

I checked our messages on our home machine, the voices of concerned friends continued to fill up the minutes. Friends we hadn't spoken with in years were checking in. Mostly we answered by e-mail.

THE NEXT NIGHT we visited my Aunt Anne and Uncle Bob in Detroit. When we made the decision to drive home, my aunt was the first person I called. We had been meaning to make the trip to Detroit anyway. I looked forward to seeing family. My uncle was sick and that visit with them in Detroit proved to be the last time I saw him—and it was the only time he met Sophie. My cousin would later tell me our visit was just what the doctor ordered.

Nursing saved me that trip. It was all about closeness. The only time I disliked nursing was in extreme heat or humidity. Yes, nursing in unfamiliar places still made me uneasy, but the act of nursing brought me great comfort. I held my baby tight. So in the back of the car, in the booth of some diner or truck stop I would nurse and the world around me seemed less horrific.

LATE AT NIGHT five days after we left Utah, we pulled into my parents' home in New Jersey. I had never been so happy to see my childhood home. My parents had bought a crib and went out of their way to take care of us.

In the morning I made Peter and Sophie go to synagogue. It was Rosh Hashanah. I had my Bat Mitzvah at that same synagogue, originally founded in part by Jewish farmers, with its relatively small congregation. We didn't have tickets but everyone made us feel at home. Sophie smiled and cooed all through the service. I knew babies could lighten up a room, but it wasn't until that week that I fully appreciated the healing power of a baby's smile.

Peter returned home the next day without me. He wanted to make sure our apartment wasn't full of dust. It wasn't. The next morning my parents drove Sophie and me into Brooklyn. We took the long way through Staten Island. Driving in the other direction were long flatbeds with the bent and twisted steel of the towers. And then there was that first glimpse of the skyline. I once heard a poet describe how absence can be stronger than presence and it was true that day looking at that empty space. Still, we were home.

Chapter 15

A Half-hour Late to a Half-hour Class *or* the Baby Formerly Known as Sophie

BEFORE WE HAD left for Utah I saw September the way I always saw September, as a new beginning. Some people make resolutions on New Year's, I tend to do it in September. Those back-to-school sales still do something to me. But I didn't feel that way after September eleventh.

All of my appointments had been canceled. I didn't reschedule them. I didn't want to go into the office again. I didn't want to take a subway or leave Sophie in Brooklyn. My emergency plan was now two pages long, soon to go on three. The write-up explained where to find the frozen milk and the formula.

I was more ambivalent about work than I previously realized. With or without September eleventh I believe the outcome would have been the same. Maybe it was because my office rent had gone up, or that the series didn't look like it was going to get renewed. Then there was that unsavory meeting with that agent. All of it left me wanting to stroll around Brooklyn with Sophie full-time. Meetings and pitches no longer appealed to me. Despite this feeling, I went through the motions of calling prospective baby-sitters. I rationalized that what I was feeling was part of the colossal post-traumatic stress we all shared in varying degrees. The key was to get back to normal, the old routine, but I was new at the mom thing. I didn't have my routine down.

THE ONLY THING on my calendar was Sophie's Music Together class. I decided if the class went well, I would sign us up for other mommy-and-me fare. Since we had already missed the first class the week before I made sure to be on time. I gave myself fifteen minutes to walk ten blocks. Of course it took me ten minutes to go from my front door to the outside stoop. That left me with five minutes. My estimations were always about fifteen minutes off. I was unable to admit to myself that the baby, stroller, and diaper bag all slowed me down. The act of packing the diaper bag alone took me about twenty minutes.

Months later I would discover the concept of always having the diaper bag ready. I recommend that you adopt this habit as soon as you return home from the hospital. Have it ready to go, four diapers, wipes, two changes of clothes for baby, a change of shirt for you. And if you don't have to pack bottles or food, it is actually the easiest your diaper bag will ever be. You'll also need a few baby toys and rattles, maybe a blanket. And of course the most important thing, a Nalgene bottle filled with water. Remember a nursing mom is always thirsty. There is nothing worse than being in a hurry to get somewhere, knowing full well you'll have to nurse the moment you arrive, and not having water. This happens to a new mom once. After that you'll always have your own water. Once you return home, pack that bag again, take out the dirty clothes, refill wipes and diapers. Of course this is an obvious suggestion, but it is the obvious stuff new moms forget. The resistance to fully embrace your new life can sometimes keep you from doing things the easy way.

I also was in the practice of nursing Sophie *before* I left the house. This, too, should be reconsidered. Later I would come to understand that even though Sophie might fuss in the stroller it was actually better to hold off nursing her. The point was to get out of the house. Once you get out your front door, you're halfway there. And when you do get to your destination, that's when you nurse.

I arrived to class fifteen minutes late. The moms were all up and dancing with their babies.

"What did I miss?" I whispered to Debra.

"The introductions," she said. Would have to catch that next time. Debra was the only mother I knew who was staying home. I met her like I met most of my mother friends, on a street corner. Debra was in another mothers' group, and like mine, most of the other mothers went back to work full-time. When she heard I was working part-time she took my phone number. She was the one who suggested taking the music class.

Since the classroom's windows were sealed shut, the room was warm and sticky, not unlike a gym locker room at the end of the day. And there were all these new moms sweating away as they shook their babies and danced in a circle. On top of that, that show-off from the mommy-and-me yoga class was there. She was even trimmer than before and wore unbelievably high-heel boots and form-fitting pants.

Don't get me wrong, I recommend that you and your baby take classes. You'll meet other new moms and usually bond with a line like, "What's with this teacher?" You'll catch a glimpse of yourself in the mirror, if you're close enough you might see the beads of sweat that form the most unflattering of mustaches. There you are, doing a jig with several colorful scarves that you're waving above your head or rattling egg shakers manically. I paid money to do stuff that would have seemed perverse even on that classic kids' TV show *The Magic*

185

Garden. Though the class was called Music Together, a more fitting name would have been *Sweating to Folk Songs*.

When I was worn out, which was about ten minutes into the class, I took a seat and used my old trick to get out of dancing. I offered Sophie my breast. That's what I did at that first class. With Sophie on my lap I sat back and caught my breath. Maybe that yoga class wasn't as advanced as I thought. If a Music Together class was going to wind me it was time to seriously rethink my physical health. At least my mothers' group would be getting together that Saturday for the first of our stroller walks. We had planned the walks months ago, but between vacations and September eleventh, we kept putting it off. Maybe the stroller walks would get me into shape.

The instructor, a petite woman with boundless energy, stood right in front of me. I had assumed my time-out to nurse would exclude me from the class, but no luck. I've never had a lap dance, but she was that close. She danced away. The thing was, Sophie loved the class. And she loved the instructor even more. If one could over-look the classroom's stuffy heat and the ridiculous sight of us moms and nannies with our bells and scarves, the class actually released a good deal of tension. It couldn't release all the tension that had built up from the car ride cross-country, from my anxieties about returning to work, and the terror of the day, but it released some.

DEBRA AND I left the class together. There was no pretense to Debra or her decision to stay home. She didn't appear to have any of the hang-ups or insecurities that I had regarding work.

"I wake up every morning and I tell my husband, 'Pinch me, am I dreaming?' I love this," she told me.

Not me. Debra suffered through my thinking out loud when I prattled on and on about finding a sitter. The fact that I hadn't

186

hired anyone for five months was evidence enough of how I actually felt, but things weren't that clear to me back then.

Aside from Debra I didn't know any other moms who were staying at home and I refused to set foot back at the breast-feeding support group. I didn't want to be known as "old waterworks." So I did what I had done in the beginning, I set about walking around the neighborhood in search of new mom friends to pick up.

AT THE PARK I saw a group of young mothers sitting at the very same table my mothers' group used to sit at. Their babies were several months younger. I walked up and introduced myself using the same old lines. How old? What's their name?

There was another Sophie in the group. Coincidence? Perhaps . . .

"She's Sophie, too," I said to the other mother as I pointed down toward Sophie's puff of black curly hair.

"She's Sophia," the mother said toward her baby. The baby could just hold her head up.

"How old?" I asked.

"Three months." The mother bent down and took her Sophia out of her stroller. When my Sophie grew up and someday donned a black beret and turtleneck, then I could see her having a preference. "Sophia," she would say. After all, I tried to jazz up my name on several occasions. I even met a woman who changed it completely from Lisa to Frankie. As an exchange student to Finland I came home with a new pronunciation, Lee-zah.

That was why I named Sophie, Sophie. I didn't know a single Sophie, not that I ever spent a second near a playground. Since none of my peers were named Sophie I saw it as unique.

I was the new kid all over again. I was an outsider to their little group so I made some nervous small talk. "You know your Sophie is the fourth one I've met. There are two in my mothers' group, and another woman at the breast-feeding support group has a Sophie."

"Her name is *Sophia*." The mother once again reminded me of her daughter's formal name. It was obvious there wasn't any leeway there. The mother was wearing a giant loose-fitting red-and-white checkered shirt. Her hair was long and pulled back tight into a ponytail. I would never have guessed she was such a stickler about her daughter's name. Then again she was the one who wrinkled her nose and said, "Ewe . . . she took a dump."

"Don't say that." Yes, I said that out loud and I believe there was a prissy shriek involved. The mother caught me off-guard with her folksy way. I had been able to go on and on about breasts and nipples but I felt strongly that little babies should make little poops. It was not my place to tell this stranger how to call her daughter's bowel movements, it just seemed that a Sophia, with that lyric dignified proper name, would not take a dump.

"Believe me, she takes dumps." The mother laid her Sophia down and began to change her diaper.

My small talk wasn't getting me anywhere so I was about to continue strolling along when another mother asked if I was staying home or heading back to work. Her name was Lonnie, she was around my height with shoulder-length red curly hair and wore a vintage *Wonder Woman* T-shirt. She was outgoing and friendlier than the other mothers at the table. Her maternity leave was running out at the end of the month.

"I'm still working part-time, but most of the mothers in my mothers' group have headed back to work. Now we are going to meet up on Saturday mornings and do a stroller walk. We're meeting this Saturday at nine in front of the bakery on Court."

"I might show up. This is Jacob. He's two months old." Her son had lots of hair and was beautiful. Lonnie's husband recently graduated law school. "With the economy slowing down he's going

188

to stay home with Jacob while he looks for work," Lonnie said. I told her about the indoor playground that was having an open house that evening. You couldn't miss all the brightly colored fluorescent posters announcing the open house. What really caught my eye for the indoor playground was the free wine and cheese. The indoor playground was also offering dozen of classes for moms and babies, and for the first week you could sit in on a "sampler" class for free.

AS PROMISED there was plenty of free wine and cheese at the open house. Peter and my mother-in-law, Nola, came along as well. It was a clean space with artwork on the walls and lots of toys in the playroom. I spotted Lonnie and she introduced me to her husband, Jeff, whom she affectionately referred to as "Mr. Mom." He told me that he was looking for a play group to hang with and if I was free we should all try and hook up. It never occurred to me that stay-at-home dads would want to be in the mothers' group. I guess I wasn't that evolved. How could I talk freely about breasts and nursing? I was polite, but unsure about a play date.

Nola was equally impressed with the facilities and bought us an annual membership, which gave us use of the indoor playground and a minimal discount on classes. We already had Music Together, but I figured I could fit one or two more classes into my schedule, even though I was working part-time.

For our first sampler, Sophie and I went to the baby movement class. There were several moms and two dads already sitting in the small colorful classroom. There was a noisy air conditioner going and one of the windows was open. Still the classroom was airless and warm. What would a mommy-and-me class be like if it wasn't airless and warm?

The teacher, a physical therapist who specialized in working with infants, was a young, well-toned woman with lots of energy. She was clear and confident in describing the class. She explained that the baby movement class was designed to give the babies the opportunity to move freely and us to learn the correct way to "walk" a baby, give the baby much needed tummy time, and understand why babies needed opportunities to explore and move on a firm surface. She explained why the floor was the best place for babies to play and that those big plastic exercise toys are great for the parents but actually do not encourage strength-building movements for babies. The information was useful.

I was happy to see that Debra and her daughter Emma had joined the class as well. And then came the introductions. The first dad introduced himself and his daughter "Sofia," with an "F." I wanted to add from the peanut gallery, "Oh, that F is really going to help, that'll keep her all unique." But in my effort to seem docile so I could make new friends I simply said, "Oh, this is Sophie too, but with a PH."

"That's our second Sophie," the teacher added, once we had gone around the room and said hello to two small Jacobs, an Olivia, a Mathew, and Emma. She began to explain what we would be doing with the babies.

The first thing we did was position our babies in crawling position. We placed their hands on the floor and their knees under their little tushies. Sophie couldn't really hold the position, her fingers curled up under her palms and her knees and thighs wanted to spread apart bringing her tummy to the floor.

"See this baby isn't ready for this yet." The instructor pointed at Sophie's hands and legs. "When this baby has more strength she'll have her fingers spread out." I took a quick glance around the room. I wasn't alone. Parents were shoving their babies into position, the babies were sliding out of position, and the parents would prop them back up again.

"He is climbing everywhere at home," one mother explained. Another mother began dragging her baby around by the hands.

"See, she loves to walk," the mother called out to the teacher.

"First things first, this is the way you walk a baby." The instructor took the baby, and instead of holding the baby's hands stretched out and up the instructor held the baby with both hands around her chest. Then she showed us how to move the baby forward. You'll see moms all the time on the toddler playground literally dragging their babies around by the hands. It's common sense, but would you really want someone to do that to you?

"Now this baby isn't really ready for this, see her toes are curling under and she isn't moving forward on her own." She handed the baby back to her overanxious mother. The grade schooler in me wanted to give the mom a look. But again, on some level I was trying to make new friends and play nice with my peer group. However, that competitiveness was there. At the end of the "sampler" class everybody wrote down their name on the sign-up sheet. It wasn't that surprising that we all wanted our babies to reach the next milestone. And having our babies assessed there in front of all the other parents raised the ante.

"Sofia with an F, love that," I rattled on to Debra as we left the class. "I've got to get this baby a nickname." In my mind Sophie was out. It was a rookie's mistake. By my own anecdotal experience it was clear, Sophie was the most ubiquitous name in Brooklyn, just as Lisa was the most ubiquitous name at NYU, and don't even get me started on the ultra common Lisa Shapiro. I know I graduated with several. Try to make a hair appointment or schedule a doctor's visit in Manhattan as Lisa Shapiro, you'll have to give your middle initial and zip code before they can pull up your file.

My poor mother had been lectured on more than one occasion on the "why couldn't you have named me something original," rant. There was always some explanation about some film called *David and*

Lisa and how at the time in 1969 Lisa was original. And now I had done to my daughter the very same thing that I myself had accused my mother of doing. The shame of it, I had yet to walk into a room with other babies and not meet at least one Sophie. It was time for a nickname no one else would have.

Piper.

I decided that Sophie's nickname was going to be Piper for no real reason or significance. I just liked the sound of it. I loved the movie *Pippi Longstocking* and this was close without being Pippi. And I decided this all by myself.

My plan was to reintroduce Sophie as Piper. At the baby movement class it was going to be Piper, it was going to be Piper whenever I introduced her, and I would call her Piper.

The next week I met up with Debra before class.

"This is Piper," I told Debra pointing down toward my stroller to the baby formerly known as Sophie.

"Piper, really, how did you come to that?"

"Just thought of it. Don't you like it?"

"Sure, if *you* like it." And off we strolled. We ran into some mommy friends of Debra's. She introduced us.

"This is Lisa and—what'shernickname?"

"It's Piper," I told the two moms. One of the babies was Lucy and the other baby was Sophia of course.

"Hi Piper." The mother of Lucy bent forward and called over to Sophie. It was odd to actually hear people call Sophie Piper. The fact that I hadn't run the nickname plan over with Peter made me feel even guiltier.

WE MEET several other people before we made it to the indoor playground. I introduced Sophie as Piper to everyone. Debra and

I were both going to attend our first official baby movement class, and as we entered the center a young woman was standing in the lobby.

"And who do we have here?" she asked us.

"This is Emma," Debra replied.

"This is Piper," I told the woman.

"Oh, Piper, I love that one." The woman confirmed my own belief that Sophie's nickname was meant to be.

AGAIN the instructor went around the room for quick introductions. When it was my turn I said, "I'm Lisa and this is Piper." No one questioned it except the father of the Sofia-with-an-F.

"I thought her name was Sophie?" he whispered over to me.

"Piper's her nickname," I told him with a mind-your-own-beeswax tone.

The instructor then told us that she began each class with a hello song, which was simple enough. We went around the circle singing, "Hello Jacob, hello Jacob, glad to see you. Hello Emma, hello Emma . . . then Hello Piper, hello Piper." It all felt so natural. Sophie looked like Piper. No more of that overused shopworn Sophie, it was now going to be Piper. The day continued and Piper made several more introductions with moms and babies.

Later that night I told Peter about Sophie's new nickname.

Peter hated the name Piper.

Perhaps I should have cleared the nickname with him sooner. After all what did he know about the commonness of Sophie? Peter wasn't out there in the mommy trenches like I was day in and day out, introduced to the flood of baby Sophies.

"I never want to hear the name Piper again. It's the worst name I have ever heard. I thought you had good taste, guess not. You didn't tell anyone her name was Piper did you?" I couldn't believe he was putting the kibosh on such a cool nickname.

"I think I told Debra," I said after a brief pause.

"Well, tell Debra her name is Sophie, you loved the name Sophie, it's such a beautiful name."

"I know that, it's just everywhere."

"So what? Did you tell anyone else her name was Piper?" Peter was hurt that Sophie had an unapproved nickname. This wasn't the reaction I anticipated.

"Not that I can remember, some moms we met, maybe at this class, but no more. Couldn't you come up with a nickname?"

"Why? I love Sophie." Peter dropped it after that. For him the whole Piper thing was over. In my mind I counted up twenty or so people I had met that day, from the park, the street, the class. Maybe everyone would forget. I planned to drop the Piper thing. Peter was free from any name hang-ups. He was a Peter not a Lisa. I didn't think men cared the way women do about names, unless you're Puff Daddy or P. Diddy.

I called Debra that night, right after Peter vetoed Piper, and left a cryptic message on her home machine. Something like, "Hi Debra, just wanted to let you know that Sophie is Sophie again. Got that? See you soon." God only knows what her husband thought of the message, but Debra understood.

And just like that Sophie was Sophie again. For nearly a week not a single mom mentioned Piper.

MY MOTHER came in to babysit. I had yet to hire a sitter. Since I needed to go to the office in the afternoon, my mother came along with Sophie and me to the baby movement class that morning.

194

Everyone took off their shoes and we all sat in a circle on the floor. I introduced my mom to the instructor.

"Okay everyone, we're all going to start with the hello song." Everyone sang, "Hello Emma, hello Emma, glad to see you, glad to see you . . ." Everyone sang hello to Mathew, Jacob, the Sofia-with-an-F, and then it was our turn. In unison everyone sang "Hello Piper, hello Piper . . ." There was no mistaking it, they were singing to us, to my Sophie.

"Wait, wait," my mother called out rather loudly for her shy self. Her eyes were wide and red. I wasn't sure at first but she was teary eyed.

"Tell them her name is Sophie." My mother was making what is sometimes called a scene. "You tell everyone right now her name is Sophie," she scolded. My mom wasn't going to let up and seeing her nearly burst into tears gave me no choice. The class stared at me.

"Everyone," I wanted to crawl under the floor mat, "I'm sorry for stopping the hello song, um . . ."

"Tell *them*," my mother implored as she wiped tears from her eyes. The nickname Piper must have hit some unknown nerve. Maybe she hated Piper Laurie?

"Her name isn't Piper." There weren't any audible gasps to this disclosure, but the class continued to look confused. "It was just a nickname."

"A terrible nickname," my mother added.

"Her name's Sophie," I told the class. The father of Sofia-with-an-F just glared at me. I admitted what he suspected all along.

"Piper was her nickname." I was in fear my mom was really going to lose it. Aside from my voice the only other sound in the room was my mother blowing her nose. "From now on her name is Sophie. Sorry about that everyone." The incredulous class tried not to look at my mother. Debra looked at me with a raised I-told-you-so eyebrow.

My mother was holding a box of tissues and periodically wiping her eyes.

"I was not prepared for *that*," my mother said to no one in particular and blew her nose again. My mother was upset because she knew and loved her granddaughter as Sophie, not Piper. The whole thing, the song, the name, all caught her off guard. At that point I could have really milked the situation with some mea culpa about Sophie's made-up and unapproved nickname Piper, but I just wanted to get on with the hello song, which had stopped in its tracks.

"Okay." The instructor tried to regain control of the class. "They don't know her name?" the instructor said softly, and then went right back into song. "Hello Sophie, hello Sophie, glad to see you, glad to see you . . ." Some of the class joined in, but it wasn't the same as before. An awkward tension filled the room, my mother continued to blow her nose into a tissue, and I could tell several parents chose not to sing, including Sofia-with-an-F's dad.

Baby movement class wasn't really the same after that. Each time we sang the Hello song I could hear a few people say "Piper." Every once in a while someone at the playground would say, "Hello Piper." Usually I let it slide. Though one time Peter came home from a stroll with Sophie and mentioned a woman said hello to Piper.

"What did you say?"

"I told her the truth, that Sophie's name was Sophie and that my wife got all insecure one day and changed her name to Piper without telling anyone."

"Did you really?"

"She was so sympathetic, she said something like 'I'm very sorry to hear that.'"

Chapter 16

Beware of Bake Sales

AT FIRST I didn't get a huge response to my babysitter e-mails. I sent them out to everyone I knew. "Looking for a babysitter, three days a week. We have two cats, an eighty-pound lab, and a three-flight walk-up. Animal lover a must." After one unsuccessful babysitter interview I learned to give full pet disclosure up front. "Are you allergic to animals?" Often the answer was yes. Or they were afraid of dogs, or didn't like buildings without elevators. Perhaps the e-mail ad wasn't as enticing as I once believed. Having spent years babysitting, I saw myself as the ideal boss. I wasn't going to ask the sitter to do light housekeeping or even walk the dog. My kitchen would hold a bounty of babysitter snacks. I guess I was in denial about our walk-up and the pets.

Several times I scheduled interviews and the women never even showed up. My mother had her own work and wasn't able to give me the same amount of babysitting as she once did. I was at the point of bringing Sophie to meetings. Things were getting desperate and I was mad at myself for putting off the issue of child care for so long.

Every time I did actually interview a seemingly nice woman something would come up. One prospective candidate could not provide a positive reference, even though she had taken care of twins for two years. Next there was a young woman from Russia who was very nice though she dressed in provocative clothing and thought the color circular from a newspaper was an appropriate teething toy for Sophie. I left Sophie and the sitter for a brief five minutes while I went to pick up a prescription. When I came back there was Sophie, newspaper dye covered her mouth and tongue.

There were ladies who were winded after the third flight of stairs and I knew it wasn't the right fit. And there was always someone who didn't care for dog slobber. Finally we found Sukie, the former sitter of Jamie from the mothers' group. Because Sukie had had to return to South America for several months, Jamie wasn't able to keep her on, but when she returned Jamie hooked us up with Sukie. She loved dogs and was only a few years older than me. She was game and knew several other sitters in the neighborhood.

Going into the office wasn't something I looked forward to. I also received word that the series wasn't going to be renewed, a fact I wasn't exactly broken up over. The series was shot on a shoestring and the economics of producing the show had changed. In many ways by the time I got around to hiring a babysitter work was slowing down. The slowdown wasn't at all unique to television production. The dot.com companies were having fire sales and friends we knew in advertising and banking were laid off. Between September eleventh and the city's recession, production jobs were no longer plentiful. I began to receive e-mails almost daily from other moms, friends of a friend, and so on. They all started the same way. "We have a wonderful babysitter, but because my company has folded or downsized, or because I was laid off . . ." In my field of work one had to constantly hustle for the next job, but suddenly that hustle wasn't the healthy challenge it once was. The first few times I left Sukie alone with Sophie I sat at my office desk and stared at my computer.

I would call Sukie several times a day just to find out how much breast milk Sophie drank, then I would pump. Most mothers I knew started solids somewhere between four and six months. Sophie was nearly six months old, but she was still sleeping through the night and nursed at her regular times. Though I knew we would be starting solids soon, she was consuming more than thirty-two ounces a day. To visualize just how much breast milk I was producing, take a look at a quart of milk. At least it was free.

NOT A MOMENT passed that fall when I didn't stop and look at Sophie and realize how lucky we were. We were some of the luckiest people on earth. My own travails in child care and working were nothing in comparison to what had happened less than a mile from our home at Ground Zero. We decided not to visit Ground Zero. However, my original mothers' group now met for our Saturday stroller walks and many of the places we strolled to were businesses affected by the attacks. We walked over the Brooklyn Bridge to Chinatown and Soho. All twelve of us, with babies and strollers, would stroll into a dim sum parlor and take a table in the back. The whole excursion was done in the spirit of adventure. Then we walked back to Brooklyn over the Manhattan Bridge, and though I didn't return home to the apartment until three in the afternoon (we had left at nine in the morning) the day left me equally exhausted and revived.

On another Saturday we all went to Boing Boing, the nursing/ maternity store in Park Slope. What I overheard at the mommy-and-me yoga class was true. There were sexy nursing bras. I bought several, all more comfortable than anything I previously owned. I also bought a sleep bra, which is an absolute must for those who need nursing pads at night. I heard about the sleep bras at the group but didn't realize what a big difference they made until I tried one on. A sleep bra is a simple invention, comfortable and seamless. There was no eyehook pressing into my back as I slept. Take it from me, before you give birth make sure you have a variety of seamless soft nursing bras and sleep bras. And you should be weary of any nursing product that needs to be hand washed. You may need to wash some items every day. My favorite bra was the soft combed-cotton number made by Japanese Weekend. It was designed in a crossover cup that you could simply pull back to nurse. It was easy to maneuver with one hand. Sophie was nearly six months old and my breasts were just beginning to feel like their old selves. My mothers' group spent quite a bit at Boing Boing. If you aren't lucky enough to have a store for nursing mothers nearby, there are many online merchants that cater to the nursing mom. My point is this: Don't wait six months to buy a comfortable nursing bra.

To my relief the bond between the mothers in the mothers' group continued to grow. We had all found solace in each other's company after the attacks, and we continued to explore as a group. Even though we no longer met during the week in the park we were all still just as close if not closer. I tried not to miss a Saturday walk and I think Peter appreciated a little alone time for himself as well. He usually went bike riding.

I COULDN'T WAIT for Halloween. It was going to be Sophie's first big holiday. I bought her a little bear costume at the Gap. It was a cute, warm slip-on bunting with a separate hat. It was perfect.

With our baby movement and nursery rhyme sing-a-long classes we were regulars at the indoor playground. The playground was going to have a party and fund-raising bake sale. Though Sophie had yet to put a single piece of food in her mouth I couldn't wait to bake for the bake sale. The great thing about having children is they give you an excuse to make all sorts of things in the juvenile vein you may otherwise opt not to.

Peter had given me *The Magnolia Bakery Cookbook* because he knew how much I loved their cupcakes and thought correctly that I would enjoy making our own. The bake sale was a perfect opportunity to try out their recipe for Traditional Vanilla Birthday Cake.

I doubled the recipe, which in my days before I learned the trick of mixing cake batter in a food processor and before I owned a Kitchen-Aid took quite a while. About a year later I would learn the true art of making cupcakes in twenty minutes. This innovation is so worthwhile that I feel it is worth breaking out of my narrative. I credit Nigella Lawson with this tip of making cake batter in a food processor. Pulse your room-temperature eggs first, then add every other ingredient and pulse. Your butter must be very soft. That's it. Take a dry $\frac{1}{4}$ measuring cup and scoop the batter into twenty-four foil cupcake cups laid out all at once on a cookie sheet. While that bakes, put all the frosting ingredients into a standing mixer, and beat until light and fluffy. Decorate using a pastry bag with large star tip, and that's it, you'll have amazing world-famous cupcakes in twenty minutes (not counting cooling time). Technique is everything. But I did not know this secret then. Somehow the whole production went on and on. I was still using cupcake tins, baking in batches, and I mixed everything with a hand mixer. By the time I brought my cupcakes to the bake sale I was proud of my work, but pooped.

I couldn't wait to see the reaction of the kids and the women manning the bake sale. I couldn't wait to hear what they would say about my cupcakes. I even went to my local bakery specifically to buy white bakery boxes to transport my cupcakes in style. Sukie took Sophie to the Halloween party at the indoor playground while I put the finishing touches on the cupcakes. With great care I walked several blocks to the center and up the flight of stairs leading to the lobby.

The table had dozens of store-bought items. I was surprised. There were individually wrapped Entenmann's pound cake, crappy cupcakes from an infamously bad neighborhood bakery, brand name cookies, and box mix brownies. The woman manning the bake sale table wore a nondescript beige sweater, large round glass frames, and short ashy hair straight and matted to her head. I handed her my box with tremendous pride. She opened the box and smiled on cue.

"These look great. I'm going to buy the whole box for five dollars," she told the woman next to her. "I have to go to a dinner party tonight and you just saved me." She laughed.

"Aren't you going to put them out? I made them for the kids."

"I just bought them." The woman dismissed me with that. I stood there stunned. There was a Halloween party going on downstairs, a party that I was already late for, a party that my daughter on her very first Halloween was enjoying with our new babysitter. I knew what I had to do, I had to find the director of the indoor playground and report the woman at once.

The director was busy telling several volunteers just where to stand. They were preparing to lead the Halloween parade around the block. Katherine, the center's director knew who I was.

"Katherine, hi I'm Lisa Shapiro, Sophie's mom."

"Yes, we're getting ready for the parade."

"I just made several dozen cupcakes for your bake sale, and the woman running the bake sale took my box and made up the price of five bucks and took them. She didn't even put them out."

"Really?" I was glad to see Katherine understood where I was coming from.

"I made them for the kids," I reiterated.

"Let me see what's going on." Katherine went over to the bake sale table. I felt sure that Katherine was going to clear up the situation and put the cupcakes out. I headed downstairs to join the party. Sophie's nursery rhyme instructor was leading the room in song. I should have joined in with the singing. I should have enjoyed the company of my mothers' group. Nora and Lonnie took the day off from work to attend the party. But instead I whispered over to my friends what had happened upstairs. I am not sure if they couldn't hear me because of the acoustic guitar and folk songs or their looks of bewilderment were because they *could* hear me.

"Can you believe that? When we go upstairs I'll give you guys a cupcake."

When we all headed upstairs my cupcakes were nowhere to be seen. The bake sale lady with her matted-down ashy hair pretended not to see me. I told Sukie to line up with Sophie for the parade and I would be there in a moment. Katherine wasn't around. I did a quick walk through the center. The open door to the coatroom revealed something familiar. On top of the steel locker-style storage closet within the coatroom was my bakery box. The bake sale lady had hidden my cupcakes in the coatroom.

Finally I saw Katherine. She was holding the door open for the kids to head outside to the parade.

"Katherine, she didn't put my cupcakes out. They are hidden in the coatroom, I just saw them." There was urgency in my voice.

"Lisa." She remembered my name. "I just spoke with her and she saw herself as paying you the highest compliment, she thought your cupcakes were so beautiful that she bought them herself. It is a fund-raiser."

"Katherine." I couldn't believe my ears. "Do you know what those cupcakes would have fetched on the open market? Those would have fetched at least eighteen dollars." I hadn't noticed the small crowd of my friends had gathered round. Debra was there, too. I didn't know her that well but on the heels of the whole Piper incident the claim

203

about my cupcakes and their price on the open market was perhaps what propelled her to take small steps back, small steps away from me. Katherine looked confused.

"That's the last time I make something for your bake sale," I said to Katherine in my you'll-be-sorry voice.

I then took my place next to Sukie and my cute little bear. The parade started, but by the time we made it around the block and back to my street I kept going, home.

"That's how bake sales get," my mother told me on the phone after listening to the whole traumatic bake sale mess. "There is always someone who brings the store-bought and buys the home-made. Trust me, there is one at every bake sale." As we discussed bake sales I realized it was one of the few times my mother has ever sounded jaded.

DEBRA TOLD ME about several moms who were getting together at a park on Wednesdays. In a continuing effort to find some more mom friends, Sophie and I went to check it out. There was Debra and Emma, several moms I had seen about the neighborhood, and, most surprising, there were two Mr. Moms. It was an egalitarian mothers' group, not just for the girls. Conversations were safe, inclusive, and had nothing to do with nursing or the other ladies' issues. Gone were the funny can-you-believe-what-my-husband-did stories or anything too personal.

I did notice quite a few dads at the playground that day. As I would later find out many were looking for work. They had been involved in new media, television, or publishing. Their wives still had their jobs. It became a familiar theme in the neighborhood. I left the park that day knowing exactly what I had to do. I pulled my mothers' group phone list out of my bag, grabbed my cell phone, and called every mom on the list.

"Next Tuesday we are all getting together at that bar on Smith Street for mommy drinking night," I said as though I received my information from headquarters. "We're all going to be there around eight o'clock, hope to see you there." Everyone was in. On Tuesday night we were all together again, my mothers' group could all allow themselves a drink and there were no Mr. Moms. It was just us, no babies. Now anyone who has read anything about nursing and alcohol knows that it is not necessarily wise to drink and nurse. And remember, I am not a lactation consultant or medical expert, I'm just a mom who knows it is okay to have a good glass of wine or light beer on the rare occasion. I always made sure to drink plenty of water as well. I do not believe in the "pump and dump." That's when you drink, pump your milk, and then throw it away. But what do I know? I do know this—the mothers' group needed a drink.

There we were. Rachel told everyone about her husband's new fish diet and how he managed to get fish oil all over her daughter's bottles. She had to hand scrub every nipple. Norma was concerned that she was being pushed out of her job at work, and Jamie wasn't sure if Oscar was going to be an only child or not. I knew I wanted to get pregnant again. The only problem was I didn't want to get pregnant until I lost more weight. I was telling everyone that once Sophie turned a year old Peter and I would start trying again. I was in mid-sentence when this tall guy with a moustache pulled a chair up to our table. He didn't even ask to sit down, plop, there he was. "Hi there. What are you ladies doing here tonight?" That was his line. Didn't he look at our ring fingers?

I couldn't help myself. After a short pause I answered, "We're all part of a breast-feeding support group."

He was stuck. It would have looked worse for him to get up and run away, though that is what he wanted to do. He didn't know what to say. He started asking us how old our babies were and we humored his questions for several minutes, until finally he wished us luck. If guys wanted to hit on the breast-feeding support group, so be it.

AROUND THE TIME Sophie was six and a half months old she woke up two nights in a row. It was time to start solids. There are different approaches to feeding an infant food. The best way to assess if your baby is ready for solids is to discuss it with your pediatrician. My pediatrician, who has worked with children for over forty years, gave me simple instructions for beginning solids with Sophie. As he directed, I bought a box of Social Tea crackers, which weren't half bad. Next I poured a little bit of breast milk over the cracker to dissolve and soften it. And with a tiny spoon I fed it to Sophie. She knew to open her mouth in anticipation of the next bite. She looked up at me with a look that said, "Where has this been?" She was a good eater.

Soon I moved on to cereal, fruits, and vegetables. I bought organic baby food and on the good advice of several moms, I purchased the baby food cookbook *Super Baby Food* by Ruth Yaron. It also included clear and simple instruction about what foods to start and when.

Social Teas can be addictive for the administering adult and one doesn't feel all that full after consuming an entire box, which can happen. I recommend making Social Tea/Nutella sandwiches. On a rainy afternoon you might be surprised how many of those yummy biscuits you can consume. So a warning, once the baby is on her way to eating solids, after that first introduction, remove the Social Teas from the home.

SOPHIE ATE baby food and nursed less and once all cookies had been banished from my kitchen, I began to drop the weight. This all happened around the time I understood how to get out of my house in less than twenty minutes. With my pre-packed diaper bag things were getting easier, faster. I no longer moved in slow motion.

Later that November I received the indoor playground's newsletter. There was a list of acknowledgments thanking all who "sent in wonderful Halloweeny treats for the bake sale." My name was included. I saved it for Sophie's baby book.

Chapter 17

Weaning

I CONTINUED with those Saturday morning walks through the fall. Lonnie, the mom I met in the park, became a regular and even Barbara, the hip yoga mom who found nursing so easy, came along. Before I had Sophie, pop culture, politics, and restaurants dotted most of my small talk. Now the conversations were consumed with discussions on child care, the office, and the housing market. It all seemed endlessly fascinating.

The women who were back at the office would preface their conversations with, "I could *never* stay home all day," or "By Sunday evening I can't wait to head back to work," or "I need adult stimulation." This was said by the members of the mothers' group with stable gigs and jobs at larger companies. One mom lost her high paying Wall Street job right after September eleventh. Now she was consulting with headhunters in her quest to "get back to work." Another mom who was a painter also worked as a graphic artist and was laid off from a children's publisher. She was looking for freelance work.

For my company to be lucrative I needed to dedicate all of my time to developing a new series. Before I had Sophie, coming home at eleven o'clock at night was the norm. Now I found it difficult to be home any later than six o'clock. There was milk to pump and freeze and a sitter to pay. The math wasn't making sense when it came to my working. I added up my take-home, subtracted the cost of child care, and came out with the most ridiculous numbers. I didn't want my company to go into debt. I had just enough money to pay for the office rent through the end of the year. In many ways the decision wasn't mine. I would have no choice but to close the Midtown office. By December I made the decision to shutter the business. I was at a crossroads. I wasn't comfortable with the notion of staying home, but in so many ways that was what I had done for the last seven months. For the first time in my life, what I wanted was not what I thought I'd wanted.

Soon after I closed my business Sukie broke the news that she could no longer work for us. She had to return home to be with her ailing mother. We would all miss her and wished her well, but the truth was, we could no longer afford a babysitter.

Those who knew me before I had Sophie said, "Not once did I ever think you would leave your work for the baby." Some told me I wasn't the stay-at-home type. Maybe I wouldn't have had the opportunity to stay home if my company was doing better. Sophie was fun to be around. She had started to crawl and babbled in the most intricate crib talk. A sure sign of true genius I told my husband. I was happiest when I was with her and most conflicted when I spoke with my former colleagues. I found myself making a case for leaving the business for a while. Though it was none of anyone's business, I would feel obliged to give the financial details of what research and development cost to create a new television series. All of it was my own tap dance.

I was surprised at how I adjusted to the slower pace. It was just Sophie and me during the day. I nursed her before she hit her hunger cry, I planned her naps and play dates, we took classes, I strolled, I cooked, I put her hair up in pigtails, and I (gasp) *enjoyed* it. The mothers' group continued the Saturday walks even through winter (our poor babies), we formed a book group, continued the drinking night to some degree, and caught a film together here and there. Life had a certain rhythm.

As slowly as time had passed when Sophie was first born, it whipped by those last few months. People told me how fast that first year goes. In the beginning I didn't believe it, but it flies. The months felt like weeks, one day I turned around and Sophie was ten months old. It was time to consider weaning.

SOPHIE HAD been favoring the right breast almost from the day she was born, but I was able to work around her preference. I would begin the first feeding in the morning on the left, offering it more than the right. Though in the last month after a minute or so she would pop off and cry for the right one. Most mothers I knew all had a winner breast. There was always one that produced more milk when pumping, or the baby always favored one over the other. They were, as one mother called them, the Loser and the Champ. Ilana suggested pumping on the left after feedings to increase the supply. I know that is what I should have done, but I was less patient with the pumping and easily slid Sophie over to the right breast instead. Which left me a little uneven, though it wasn't obvious to anyone else. At least no one said anything, not even Peter.

There had been one mom at our support group who nursed her daughter exclusively on one breast. It produced enough. And one mother I met in the park who nursed her twins told me how each baby would be fed solely on one breast for an entire day, then the next morning she would switch, thus keeping the production somewhat even. It was amazing the methods and tricks women came up with to even out their breasts. In some ways Sophie had been weaning herself off my left breast for some time.

Sophie had become busy with the business of life. Nursing was no longer her top priority. She could say Mama, Dada, doggie, and cheese. We were very proud of the latter. Each day she seemed to take on a new word. She applauded herself, often clapping her hands together. We talked and sang to her constantly. Sophie opened and shut her hands when we sang "Twinkle Twinkle Little Star." She was cruising on everything. Cruising is when a baby holds onto furniture or the rail of their crib and walks alongside. They aren't ready to walk on their own, but they can move quite fast when holding onto furniture. While Sophie was playing I called Jan, a friend from the mothers' group, to make plans for a play date. A quick word about play dates. In that first year your darlings won't really notice other babies much less play with them. They may smile and grab at other babies, but they are still too young to play dress up. They are important and of course help in socializing your baby. But mostly they are for you.

Without warning, Sophie walked. I told Jan I would have to call her back. As Sophie marched toward me, she took strong, definitive strides. I grabbed the video camera. It's important to have your video camera ready to go at all times. We were in the good habit of having it loaded with tape and fully charged. So I caught Sophie's second set of steps. There she was, eleven months old and walking.

From the moment Sophie stood up in the middle of the living room and walked, she never really sat down again. She walked and walked. We had successfully baby-proofed most of the apartment, but there was always something she would get into. One of the cheapest and most important things we did was to install those outlet plates. The other kind, those plastic buttons, are also safe. The problem was not that Sophie couldn't remove them, but we couldn't either. At least not without breaking a nail. We put a foam pad around our bench in the living room and had a retractable gate for the kitchen. It was a durable white mesh gate and retracted into a neat roll—one of the best baby things we've ever purchased.

I also purchased sippy cup tops for her Avent bottles. Sophie had yet to master the straw and though she preferred the wide silicone nipples over the non-drip spout, she was old enough to make the switch. I took breast milk out of the freezer, defrosted it, put it in the sippy cup, packed that in the diaper bag, and headed out to the park.

At the park I did something I had never done before. I pulled out the bottle and said to Debra, who mind you never asked, "It's breast milk. I am in the process of weaning her." Wasn't I defensive at giving Sophie a bottle in public? So much of my identity had been wrapped up with nursing. I was unsure about who I was going to be as a mom once I weaned Sophie. I did know this, and I didn't want her to someday soon ask for it. I once saw a toddler point to her mother's chest and call out, "Titties," and I knew that wasn't for me.

There are many traditions, methods, and philosophies when it comes to weaning. There are people who believe abrupt weaning is best. I have heard stories of mothers who left town for the week or weekend to wean their children. In some cultures, women were known to rub coco powder on their breasts and tell their toddlers that it was feces. Gradual weaning happens over weeks and months and eases the child from the breast. If it is done at the right pace the act of weaning can be a mutual desire of child and mother. I knew I wasn't going to do the coco method, so I decided to wean Sophie gradually.

Things that are sometimes hard-won are difficult to give up, but that wasn't the case for me. After nursing became easy I feared I would want to nurse for years, but I was ready to wean. I spoke with Ilana and other mommy friends about how to achieve this by Sophie's first birthday.

I wanted my breasts back. I daydreamed about underwire lace bras. There were push-ups to purchase and dresses to wear. Summer was a few months away. Perhaps I would fit into my Lilly Pulitzers again. There was more weight to lose, and losing it can be easier once you wean. Peter and I wanted another baby. I needed to get back in shape. So there I was with that sippy cup of breast milk in the park.

It wasn't something Sophie loved. She chewed on the spout, took a few efficient sucks and pushed it away. Things went like that. Then I ran out of the frozen breast milk. I wasn't up for pumping more. Since Sophie was nearly a year, I weaned her to diluted drinkable yogurt and then onto organic whole milk. I dropped a single feeding about every two weeks.

By her first birthday we were down to three feedings a day, once in the morning, once in the afternoon, and right before bed. The truth about your baby's first birthday party is it is your coming out party. "It's been a year, ladies and gentlemen, let's see if she's still fat." I wasn't fat. I was about eight pounds shy of where I was before I was pregnant. I wanted to lose more, but I no longer hated how I looked. Another milestone.

I loved planning the party. We were low-key about Sophie's baby naming, which we had at our synagogue a month before. So we saw her birthday as the perfect excuse to go ridiculously overboard, especially since Sophie shared her birthday with Peter and his father. We had it in a loft, which overlooked the Brooklyn Bridge and Manhattan skyline.

Yes, a hundred guests was overkill. I ordered something like fifty silver Mylar balloons. The cotton candy machine, clown, and Elmo weren't required, and having the whole event catered with an open bar wasn't a complete necessity, but at the time I felt they were. The mothers' group was there and several of our little ones were walking around. Rachel's Sophie gave my Sophie a hug.

All of the guests had an opportunity to pose for a picture with Elmo, and most did. I wore a tight denim skirt and a fitted white shirt. It was one of the first times I felt pretty again. There are no photos

213

of me from Sophie's first year hanging in our home. There are many of Sophie, but none of me with one exception; our family portrait with Elmo is prominently displayed.

THE WEEK before Mother's Day my mom and I brought Sophie to visit my grandmother in Maine. It was great having all four generations of mothers and daughters together. I was down to two feedings. She had dropped the afternoon one right after her party.

Since we arrived in Maine, Sophie was disinterested in the evening feeding at that point. The morning was the only one left. With Sophie walking, she had so many people to see and places to go. There was no point in forcing a feeding. I thought she would hang onto that morning feeding for months to come. She was groggy and hungry when she woke. She wasn't a little baby anymore. She was over twenty pounds, but I still used my pillow. It kept my back straight. Yes, I used "My Brest Friend" pillow for the entire year. Unlike several ladies in my mothers' group, I was never able to nurse while lying down, I could go without my pillow but preferred not to, and for the sake of comfort and habit I kept to that belly-to-belly position.

On Mother's Day Sophie woke up hungry. I did what I had done for the last year.

I took Sophie and placed her across my lap on my nursing pillow. As I attempted to bring her in I felt resistance as I moved her head into my breast. She looked up at me, smiled, and shook her head no. Sophie knew that shaking one's head side to side indicated no. It was all very polite and I went with it.

I took her off my lap, changed her diaper, dressed her and took her downstairs for breakfast. I handed her a sippy cup full of milk and she drank it.

Were we really through? That night after I put Sophie to bed I decided that the next morning I would once again attempt to nurse Sophie, just to be sure, just to be certain that she was in fact done. Sophie woke the next morning and I did my same routine. I brought her again onto my nursing pillow and attempted to latch her on just as I'd always done. This time Sophie was frustrated. She burst into tears and shook her head no again. Sophie stared up at me with the most perplexed look on her face. Her face wore her thoughts, "Hey what are you doing? Why are you trying to stick that nipple into my mouth, you freak? I told you no thanks." I immediately sat her up and she stopped crying. It just wasn't for her anymore. We were done. I e-mailed the gals in the mothers' group, "We've weaned."

Several of the moms wrote back words of support, like "Soon you'll have another baby and you'll nurse that one." Rachel welcomed me, "to the other side." I wasn't sad, I wasn't depressed. I felt freed.

SOPHIE WAS a toddler now. There was a novelty fish at my parents' place in Maine. It looked like a mounted prized bass, but when you pushed a button it sang, "Take Me to the River." Sophie loved that fish. She would push the button and dance. Her dancing consisted of Sophie bending slightly forward, she would put both hands on her thighs, and shake her tiny butt.

We were on to the next stage. She was no longer my nursling. She was a toddler who loved to dance to a novelty fish. I wouldn't have it any other way.

215

Chapter 18

In Sync with the Universe

RIGHT AROUND the time I weaned Sophie I got my first official letter from my insurance company denying all coverage for my visits with the lactation consultants. I had even included a letter from my midwife explaining the need for the lactation consultants because of my difficulties and Sophie's bout with jaundice. They would not even pay a partial sum. I wrote a letter stating how research had shown breast-fed babies are generally sick less often than formula-fed babies and that that in turn would cost the insurance company less. I made an official complaint to their grievance board and even appealed their first decision, which I lost. By June, a year and two months since I had Sophie, I received the final verdict. They wouldn't pay a dime.

Soon after I received a package from my insurance company. No they hadn't changed their mind and it wasn't a check, instead they sent me a thin booklet entitled "A Guide to Baby Massage."

I'M NOT SURE if the weight drops off your body the second you wean, but I do know that I was no longer famished. Food wasn't something I was hungry for all the time. I went back to three meals a day instead of my nursing mom's five. While I was nursing, I became the water-drinking equivalent of a chain smoker. I couldn't leave my house without a Nalgene bottle full of cold Brita water. Now hours could pass before I would have the urge to drink a glass of water. And so my weight did drop. And where the weight seemed to drop first was my breasts, they shrunk. First they shrunk to their pre-baby size, and then for the hell of it, they seemed to get even smaller. My pre-pregnancy bras had a cup size full of air. I wore stretchy soft cups and even purchased a Wonder Bra with padding. Smaller breasts didn't seem that bad to me. I know some women who are obsessed with their cup size, perhaps it's because we live in the age of implants, but I'll take small, soft, and round over large and engorged any day. Some of my old size-eight clothes were finally fitting, and the size ten looked loose. I was rid of my new mom's ass.

Several of my friends from the mothers' group had recently weaned as well so we made plans for a girls' night out. And with my newfound independence and ability to drink alcohol at will, I planned to get fairly tipsy.

I HAD WANTED to lose weight, not just because I was vain, but because I wanted to get pregnant again. Peter and I had talked about having children spaced within two years of each other. Since I was home and since we had all the stuff, the clothes, the gear, and even a few tiny diapers, why not? When Sophie was eight and nine months old I remember thinking that I wasn't ready, but by the time she was eleven months I leafed through a maternity catalog. Because I had taken Clomid to conceive Sophie, I thought we would give ourselves a year to try for another one. My midwife told me that in her experience she had seen several women who had Polycystic Ovarian Syndrome who needed help getting pregnant the first time, but had no trouble conceiving their second child. And just to make sure all was up and running, I scheduled my yearly visit with Suzanne my midwife.

Though my breasts had shrunk they still felt slightly lumpy. I avoided touching them and I knew not to let the water from my shower beat down on them either. The last thing I wanted was to stimulate milk production. I believed my breasts would even out over time and I was just experiencing the normal effects of weaning.

I told Suzanne I had recently weaned and was discussing my desire to try and get pregnant when she began to look over my file for my family's breast cancer history. She examined my breasts again and told me that because my grandmother and great-grandmother had had breast cancer she wanted to be on the safe side and schedule an appointment for me with a breast specialist. "Most likely the lumps in your breast are because you recently weaned, but you do have a history of breast cancer in your family and I would rather be overly cautious in this situation."

Breast cancer?

I called Peter at his office. "Could you meet me for lunch?" I explained Suzanne's concern and we called my father-in-law at his hospital. I had been through too much with my breasts in the last year. Was I a fool? Were all of my problems nursing a result of something else? Something wrong? What if nursing had disguised my true condition?

When Peter spoke with his dad he told us not to worry, that he knew an excellent breast specialist and I was able to get an appointment later that week. I didn't feel up for mommy drinking night, so I bailed. My father-in-law told me several times not to worry, but the very idea of breast cancer was enough to keep me up for the better part of two nights.

My father-in-law met me at the breast specialist's office so he could watch Sophie while I had my appointment. Sophie loved seeing her Papa and he read to her from various women's magazines in the waiting room.

The doctor was a lovely woman in her fifties. She was a renowned breast surgeon and she insisted I call her Diane. "Okay, let's take a look. I am almost certain everything is fine, but let's do an examination." She examined my breasts and went on and on about my father-in-law.

"He is just wonderful, everyone thinks so." And with that she pushed down hard on my breast and just like that milk shot up Old Faithful–style right into the doctor's face.

"Oh, did that get you? I'm so sorry," I said as she grabbed a tissue.

"No, no it's just milk, that's what I thought. Believe me that's nothing." She didn't elaborate, nor did I ask her to. "Okay, get dressed and we'll talk in my office." I got dressed and took a seat in her office. I was on auto-pilot.

"So everything's okay. Some women have milk in their breasts for as long as two years. I've seen that in patients."

"Have you seen women who after they weaned discovered a problem?"

"Yes, I have seen some real nightmares, but that's not your case. Okay, good luck with the baby."

I used to wear pads twenty-four hours a day so I wouldn't leak a drop in public. I used to think that was the nightmare scenario. Here

219

I had squirted a renowned doctor directly in the face with breast milk and it was one of the better things that had happened to me.

WITH MY clean bill of health, I told Peter it was time to make another baby. Now here's the thing about weaning, and this may just be my experience, but I believe right after I weaned I was very fertile. I got pregnant the first time we tried. I joked that I was carrying the Messiah. Several moms I knew had similar experiences, so consider yourself warned.

At the next mommy drinking night I drank seltzer.

THE IDEA of having two children was overwhelming, but I would have some time to prepare. In the meantime, there were parks to play at and museums to visit. I could give Sophie a sippy cup of milk as I pushed the stroller. It enabled me to multitask. I didn't have to stop what I'm doing to feed my daughter, and I'm not entirely sure that was a good thing.

I never loved nursing. Still, I learned to appreciate those calm quiet moments when time seemed to stop and I nursed my baby. The beauty of it was in the let-down of milk, the skin-on-skin contact, and that sense of being in sync with the universe.

Epilogue

Cranks, Hot Mamas, and Sherpas

I RECENTLY attended another open house for the indoor playground. I hadn't been by that often, not since that bake sale fiasco. But I'm a sucker for free food and it was that sort of gathering. I also felt it was time to put what happened to my cupcakes and me in the past.

My seven-month-old son Eben was asleep in my New Native Baby sling and my daughter, Sophie, nearly two and a half, was playing with the pink plastic kitchen in the playroom. For all the time I put in strolling about the neighborhood I recognized few faces. Most of the people mingling looked like new parents. I noticed several new moms with young babies talking amongst themselves. They were the bizzaro version of my mothers' group. There was one mom who had long curly hair like Rachel, another who wore the same eyewear as Lonnie, and there was a mom who reminded me of me, perhaps it was because she was doing all of the talking. They were all going on about how great the indoor playground was and which classes they were going to take. Part of me, the hey-I'm-a-mother-of-two-I-know-everything part, wanted to waltz up to them and warn them, saying something saucy like, "Yeah, but don't bake anything for the bake sale." But I stopped myself. I am a recovering know-it-all and recognize when not to interrupt the deluded. In the hierarchical world of moms, they were freshman and somewhere along the way I graduated from senior to crank.

Then there are days when it all works for me and I feel the faint sensation of being a hot mama. The kids sleep through the night, I like my shoes, my hair, and all the superficial trappings that make me feel good and happy. But there is the crank in me. It makes me say things like, "Newborns are wasted on new moms." I have crank friends. One told me that she loved her children most when they're sleeping. When Sophie and Eben get sick, our apartment turns into the Dimetapp equivalent of a crack den, with little infant-dose syringes everywhere. And my sense of time isn't what it used to be, though expired coupons are evidence that it has indeed passed. I am the secretary for my babysitting co-op and keep track of everyone's points on a spreadsheet. I've had my weird nightmares with *The Wiggles*, which left me unable to see them live in concert the same way again. I secretly hope Murray will come out into the audience and grab my hand, but I am unwilling to make the requisite banner.

The backpack carrier for Eben is actually called Base Camp, that's the model name. And I look like I'm leaving base camp when he's in that thing. With two kids in two years I sometimes think what I've really become is a Sherpa. That's what I am when I push my double Maclaren Rally Twin up a hill or shove it through the doors of my local coffee shop.

I looked over at those new mothers at the indoor playground with the most bittersweet of longing, the most wistful of thoughts slipping through my mind. Ah, I was you. I was that once-in-a-lifetime thing, a new mom. Savor it all for that early adventure is brief.

222

On most days when I notice a new mom struggling with her carrier or stroller I have a glad-that's-not-me moment. The urge to pass along unsolicited advice is no longer there. Though sometimes I do the appropriate thing and yell, "It gets easier," from the safety of my moving car.

But looking over at those new moms that night I was aware of exactly what I felt. It was envy.

Acknowledgments

THIS BOOK would not exist without the belief and vision of my editor Ann Treistman. She was always available and guided me with her deft touch. I would not have been able to write the book without my husband, Peter Steinberg, who watched our babies on countless evenings and weekends. He also happens to be the world's best literary agent, and many thanks to JCA Literary Agency. I would have no story to tell without Ilana Taubman and Laura Best-Macia of Wellcare, Inc., who taught me how to feed my daughter. I owe so much to Wendy Shanker, who kept me honest and read every draft. I am grateful to Eliza Byron and all the great people at The Lyons Press for their commitment and enthusiasm for my book.

Many thanks to my family and friends for their unwavering support and generosity: My parents Lucy and Mike, my sisters Anne and Amy, my in-laws Nola and Harry, and also Dara and Nick—I am so lucky to have you all. Stacey Simon, who came into our lives right when we so needed her and made it possible for me to do my work. And I don't know where I would be if not for the inspiring and funny women of my mothers' group who suffered me gladly and taught me a great deal—Michele, Emily, Kristen, Liz, Christine, Judy, and especially Meredith Murphy and Ann LoBue for their early reads of my proposal. I am thankful for Long Island College Hospital's Breast-feeding Support Group. And also to all the wonderful moms I've met along the way.

I will always be indebted to Lucy Grealy and her workshops and to my grandmother Frances B. Wood, who loved books.

Bibliography

Appel, Jennifer and Allysa Torey, 1999. *The Magnolia Bakery Cookbook*. New York: Simon & Schuster.

Eisenberg, Arlene, et al. 1996. *What to Expect the First Year*. New York: Workman Publishing.

Eisenberg, Arlene, et al. 1996. *What to Expect When You're Expecting*. New York: Workman Publishing.

Huggins, Kathleen and Linda Ziedrich. 1994. *The Nursing Mother's Guide to Weaning*. Boston: The Harvard Common Press

Huggins, Kathleen. 4th Edition, 1999. *The Nursing Mother's Companion*. Boston: The Harvard Common Press.

La Leche League International, 6th Edition, 1997. *The Womanly Art of Breastfeeding*. New York: Plume.

Lawson, Nigella. 2001. *How To Be A Domestic Goddess: Baking and the Art of Comfort Cooking.* Great Britain: Hyperion.

Mason, Diane and Diane Ingersoll. Revised Edition,1997. *Breastfeeding and the Working Mother.* New York: St. Martin's Griffin.

Tupler, Julie and Andrea Thompson. 1996. *Maternal Fitness.* New York: Fireside.

Resources

There are many sites and stores that cater to the nursing mother. Here is my short list.

LACTATION CONSULTANTS

International Lactation Consultant Association
1500 Sunday Dr., Ste. 102
Raleigh, NC 27607
919-861-5577
www.ilca.org
info@ilca.org

You can search through its Web site to find a lactation consultant in your area.

Wellcare, Inc.
Breastfeeding Services and Lactation Centers
212-696-9256
888-baby-234

These centers serve the New York City area only. Wellcare has wonderful lactation consultants and runs support groups.

BREAST PUMPS AND SUPPLIES

Medela, Inc.
Breastfeeding National Network
800-TELL-YOU
www.medela.com

Medela makes excellent pumps to rent and own, along with parts, bras, breast shells, footstools, special-needs feeding supplies, and many other breast-feeding products. Call to find nursing bras, a breast-feeding specialist in your area, and where to rent a breast pump.

The Pump Station
2415 Wilshire Blvd.
Santa Monica, CA 90403
877-842-7867
www.pumpstation.com
info@pumpstation.com

This is the ultimate store for nursing mothers. It has everything including a huge line of nursing bras and clothes, nursing pillows, pumps, pump supplies, baby clothes, and a large selection of books.

It also holds classes and has lactation consultants and support groups. Right now it serves only the Los Angeles area.

NURSING PILLOW

My B*rest* Friend Nursing Pillow
www.zenoffproducts.com

The Zenoff Products Web site lists where to buy "My B*rest* Friend" both online and in stores. I recommend a quick online browse because prices vary. I've seen "My B*rest* Friend" pillows go for as much as $54 at a baby store and for as little as $32 online.

BABY CARRIERS

BabyBjörn
www.babybjorn.com

Almost every baby store I have shopped at carried the ubiquitous BabyBjörn carrier. You can also order a catalog from its Web site. I have met women who have had success nursing their babies while they carried them in this carrier.

The New Native Baby Carrier
800-646-1682
www.newnativebaby.com
I used the BabyBjörn with Sophie but became a true convert to this sling with Eben. The smooth lightweight cotton fabric holds up well, it comes in all different colors including black, and it is seamless with no rings, belts, or snaps. I was able to nurse my son on several occasions while wearing him in the sling.

MOTHER TO MOTHER SUPPORT

La Leche League International
1400 N. Meacham Rd.
Schaumburg, IL 60173
800-La-Leche
www.lalecheleague.org

You can find a support group through its Web site, by calling the 800-number, or by checking with your local hospital.

NURSING CLOTHES

Motherwear
800-950-2500
www.motherwear.com

Motherwear has a wide variety of nursing bras, along with sleep bras and many other clothes with flaps and pull-away panels. You'll also do well browsing the Web; there are many sites that carry nursing bras and like.

PROVISIONS (IN ORDER OF NECESSITY)

Jacques Torres Chocolate
66 Water Street
(Between the Brooklyn & Manhattan Bridges)
Brooklyn, New York 11201
718.875.9772 phone
www.mrchocolate.com
info@mrchocolate.com

I didn't discover this amazing chocolate until I was nursing my second child, but I quickly made up for lost time.

Bon Bons Chocolatier
319 Main Street
Huntington, NY 11743
631-549-1059
www.bonbonschocolatier.com
contact@bonbonschocolatier.com

If you can, visit their store. It's exactly what a chocolate shop should be.

See's Chocolates
1-800-347-7337
www.sees.com

Their bridge mix is the best in the world.

Termini Bros.
1523 South 8th Street
Philadelphia, PA 19147
800-882-7650
www.termini.com

The make-your-own cannoli kit from Termini Brothers bakery is one of the best ever new mother gifts.

Artie's Deli
2290 Broadway (at 83rd)
New York, NY 10024
212.579.5959
www.arties.com
info@arties.com

They send amazing care packages for "displaced" New Yorkers anywhere in the country.

Taste of Texas Barbecue
403 Potomac St.
Taylor, TX 76574
512-352-5624
www.tasteoftexasbarbecue.com

My entire family lived on this barbecue for days after my son was born. It was truly a lifesaver.

About the Author

Lisa Wood Shapiro is a writer and an Emmy-winning filmmaker whose work has appeared on PBS, A&E, Nickelodeon, Noggin and elsewhere. She studied nonfiction writing with the late Lucy Grealy and the poet Thomas Lux.

Lisa lives in Brooklyn, New York with her husband and two children.